REAL LIFE 101:

A GUIDE TO STUFF THAT ACTUALLY MATTERS

DEREK AVDUL
&
STEVE AVDUL

 GALT INDUSTRIES LLC

Library of Congress Control Number: 2003195196

ISBN 0-9747287-0-5

Manufactured in the United States of America

This publication contains the opinions and ideas of the authors and is intended to provide helpful and informative material on the subject matter covered. It is sold with the understanding that the authors and the publisher are not engaged in rendering legal, accounting, or other professional advice. If legal advice or other expert assistance is required, the services of a competent professional should be sought.

The authors and publisher specifically disclaim any responsibility for any liability, loss or risk, personal or otherwise, which is incurred as a consequence, direct or indirectly, of the use and application of any of the contents of this book.

Product or brand names used in this book may be trademarks or registered trademarks. For readability, they may appear in initial capitalization or have been capitalized in the style used by the name claimant. Any use of these names is editorial and does not convey endorsement of or other affiliation with the name claimant. The publisher does not intend to express any judgment as to the validity or legal status of any such proprietary claims.

Cover design by Derek Avdul & Steve Avdul

Published by Galt Industries LLC, Post Office Box 2886, Hollywood, CA 90078
www.galtindustries.com

10 9 8 7 6 5 4 3

ACKNOWLEDGEMENTS

The authors would like to thank the following people for their assistance, guidance, input, and overall help and support in creating this book. We could not have done it without you. Many thanks to Don and Linda Avdul, Jay Avdul, Brett Dallesandro, Ro Kolakowski, Mary Trautman, Frank Hajdu, Kent Erickson, Galt Industries, 6th Street Consulting, Sudie White and the entire team at Central Plains Book Manufacturing.

We also appreciate the contribution of many of our friends and associates who made introductions, pointed us in the right direction, and generally helped in any way they could.

DEDICATION

To Mom and Dad for a lifetime of love and support.

CONTENTS

INFORMATION BOXES

abc...

INTRODUCTION

*R*eal Life 101: A Guide To Stuff That Actually Matters. What is the stuff that actually matters? Basically it's the *practical* things adults living on their own in the United States need to know in order to function in society. It's not about answers to questions regarding career, relationships, or spirituality. Those topics are beyond the scope of this book. *Real Life 101* addresses stuff like renting an apartment, buying a car, managing your money, and taking care of yourself—the tasks that make up the *everyday living* part of life. These are not exactly Earth-shattering topics but try getting along in this world without paying attention to them. It's possible but certainly makes life a lot more difficult.

Like many people, you're probably thinking to yourself, "But I already know how to do all this stuff." Do you? Okay, then here are a few questions. Based on your income, how much should you be spending on an apartment each month? What's the difference between an HMO, a PPO, and a POS? Given a four-year loan and a 7% interest rate on a $25,000 car, how much is your monthly payment going to be? What about comparing leasing versus buying a car, which is the better option? Should you get a debit card, a charge card, or a credit card? Hmm, maybe you don't quite know all of these things. That's okay; this book is here to help.

In school you learned how to calculate the area of triangle, read a little Billy Shakespeare, and found out that Abe Lincoln was the 16th President of the United States. Good knowledge if you're ever a contestant on *Jeopardy!* but not particularly helpful with life's day-to-day tasks. That's where this book comes in. *Real Life 101: A Guide To Stuff That Actually Matters* covers all the information you need to know for life in the real world.

This book tackles issues such as creating a budget, renting an apartment, moving, shopping for a car, understanding health insurance, managing your finances, and staying organized. Each chapter is designed to address one specific issue, or in some cases one aspect of an issue, and present the topic in as straightforward a manner as possible. Individual chapters break everything down and offer tips and helpful hints along the way. Information boxes provide examples and checklists related to the topic to ensure that nothing is overlooked when you are making your decisions. This book arms you with valuable information and gives you the tools needed to make some of life's decisions simpler and some of life's little challenges easier.

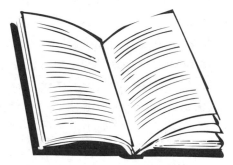

HOW TO USE THIS BOOK

An often-neglected topic with books such as *Real Life 101: A Guide To Stuff That Actually Matters* is how to use them in the most effective manner. First, let's cover what this book is not. It is not a career, relationship, or spiritual guide nor does it address any interpersonal or professional issues. Also, it is not a novel that you would sit down and read cover-to-cover.

Instead, this book assumes that you already have a job and are earning income and concentrates on simplifying your life when it comes to the issues of your home, car, health, and finance. Each chapter is designed to take the hassle out of life's everyday tasks, shorten the time it takes to do them, provide helpful hints and insight to "uncomplicate" these issues, and generally tell you what you need to know to get things done quickly and efficiently.

The best way to use this book is on a chapter-by-chapter or topic-by-topic basis. Before making the decision regarding an apartment, car, health insurance, or your finances, examine the chapter that addresses that area. Read through the relevant chapters to increase your knowledge of the subject *in advance* of starting the actual process. Review the information boxes to understand the key factors you should consider in making your decision. Additionally, use the helpful companion to this book, *Real Life 101: The Workbook* to create your own checklists and templates that you can fill out while making each choice.

In short, use this book as a preparation tool. There is no need to study the chapter on leasing a car if you won't be leasing one until a year from now. Don't get overwhelmed by trying to master all the information on every topic at one time. Think of the book as a series of information booklets that you can use and review when confronted with a specific decision.

Real Life 101: A Guide To Stuff That Actually Matters was created through many years of confronting each situation, making mistakes, and learning along the way. You shouldn't expect to be an expert on every topic. Just use the information included in each chapter to your advantage as that issue becomes relevant in your life. By so doing, you can avoid many common errors and make informed, sound decisions in life on the stuff that actually matters.

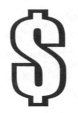

CHAPTER 1
BUDGETING

C hapter One: Budgeting. Yikes! What a scary topic with which to begin. For many, the thought of creating a budget sounds about as painful as a trip to the dentist but it doesn't have to be. As you'll see with each topic covered in this book, it's all about simplifying life not complicating it. So it goes with budgeting. Don't worry. You won't be counting pennies on a weekly basis or foregoing the movies on Saturday night because you bought an extra loaf of bread on Thursday. But you do need to adopt the most basic of budgets or at least be familiar with the concept to ensure you live within your means and enjoy life as much as possible.

This book covers topics ranging from renting an apartment to buying a car to selecting proper healthcare to managing your finances. Well, all of this starts by creating a simple budget. It's quite difficult and potentially dangerous to start off renting a place and buying a car without first determining how much you can realistically afford to spend on these items. By developing a simple budget you can "ballpark" how much money you can pay for your two largest monthly expenses. And for many, credit cards can also be a third major monthly expense.

People aged 24-34 spend on average $641 per month on rent and utilities

So let's get to it. The Big Three: Rent, Car, Credit Card. For most Americans, regardless of age, housing costs, transportation, and debt service (fancy ways of saying rent, car, and credit card) are the largest monthly expenses and the expenses over which they actually have the most direct control. Let's face it, food and healthcare are basic necessities and most people can't really change how much these items cost every month. Health insurance is what it is and unless you're willing to radically change your diet, there isn't a whole lot you can do to dramatically lower your food bill.

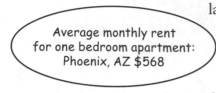

Average monthly rent for one bedroom apartment: Phoenix, AZ $568

That brings us back to The Big Three. The funny thing is, although all three of these expenses are well within most people's control, they almost never think of them as expenses that can be managed. Typically, people pay the rent, the car payment, the credit card bills, and then think, "How much money do I have left?" Well it's true, once you've moved in, bought a car, and run up the credit cards, these expenses suddenly are "fixed" every month. So let's take a moment and deal with them before they're etched in stone.

Although everyone has a slightly different opinion as to exactly how much each of these expenses should cost you every month, a good rule of thumb is outlined in Box 1. Your gross income is how much you make before taxes and other items are taken out of your paycheck (i.e., your salary of $24,000 per year or your wage of $12.00 per hour).

BOX 1: BIG THREE EXPENSES

Recommended % of Gross Income:

Rent	25% - 30%
Car Payment	10% - 15%
Credit Card Payments	0% - 5%

Rent should be approximately 25% to 30% of gross income, car payment in the range of 10% to 15% of gross income, and although the ultimate goal is 0%, credit card debt should cost you no more than 5% of your gross income. In total, this means that at the low end of the range, these three items should be approximately 35% of gross income but at the high end no

The starting price for a 2004 Honda Accord DX Sedan is $15,900

more than 50%. Again, opinions vary, but a combined 40% for The Big Three is a number that should maximize your comfort level in terms of housing and transportation without breaking the bank.

Remember that these numbers are not absolute minimums or maximums; they are merely guidelines to help you plan what may be best for you. Assume you make $24,000 a year and spend 25% on housing, 10% on your car, and buy a few CDs and therefore spend 5% on credit cards each month. In this case you'd spend $500 a month for rent, $200 a month for your car, and $100 a month on credit card debt. Don't forget that these three items work together. If you tend to spend a little extra on the credit card, perhaps you should shop for a less expensive car. On the other hand, if your car is extremely important to you, then spend a little more on your ride but see what you can do about renting a less expensive place. Think about what you can realistically afford *before* you sign the apartment lease and *before* you buy the new car.

You can make the whole "budgeting" process a heck of a lot easier if you haven't dug yourself a deep hole by overspending on The Big Three. Take your annual gross income, divide it by 12 to get your monthly income, and then multiply that by the suggested percentage guidelines and you'll have a quick

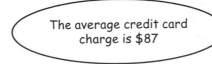

The average credit card charge is $87

feel for approximately how much you should be spending each month on these expenses.

Okay, you've done a quick "back-of-the-envelope calculation" with regard to how much you can afford for rent, car, and credit cards, but what about the rest of the money? Where does it go? Let's start back at the top and work down through the standard monthly expenses. Box 2 provides an example based on earning $24,000 and the recommended percentages for spending on each category. As already mentioned, The Big Three account for

BOX 2: HOUSEHOLD EXPENSES

	Annual	Monthly	Percent
Gross Income	$ 24,000	$ 2,000	100%
Rent	($ 6,000)	($ 500)	25%
Car Payment	($ 2,400)	($ 200)	10%
Credit Card Payment	($ 1,200)	($ 100)	5%
Taxes	($ 6,000)	($ 500)	25%
Net Available Income	$ 8,400	$ 700	35%

Other Expenses to Remember:
Utilities, Insurance, Food, Clothing, Entertainment, Savings

the first 40% of expenses and taxes can quickly eat up 25% or more. Just like that, you've blown through two-thirds of your paycheck. Welcome to Adulthood!

The real question is what to do with the remaining third. Well, before you're off buying the latest plasma screen TV, remember a few other expenses that rear their ugly heads. Don't forget about your monthly utilities such as phone, cell phone, power, cable, Internet, and the like. Of course there is also health insurance, car insurance, gas, and car maintenance. Oh yeah, you haven't eaten a thing yet either so you'll have to go to the 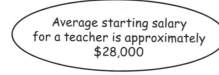 grocery store and buy some food. And unless you live in a nudist colony, you'll need to buy some clothes along the way as well. Finally, you've still got to entertain yourself (e.g., go to the movies, eat at a restaurant, attend a concert or sporting event). And if there is any money left over, saving for a rainy day is always a fantastic idea.

The point is this: writing down how much you spend each month compared to how much you make is not a particularly fun topic. But spending a little time thinking about your major expenses and using the household expenses template included in *Real Life 101: The Workbook* will make it much easier to manage the smaller expenses down the road.

Use the information included in this chapter to assist you in determining how much you can afford to spend on The Big Three. Remember, even though the table may indicate that you can spend $500 per month on rent, if you find a great apartment for $375, that's an extra $125 to cover your other expenses, pay down some credit card debt, and maybe even start saving some money! Keeping in mind all the expenses that constitute your normal monthly spending pattern will put you in control of your finances and in a position to maximize your paycheck as well as your life.

Median wage for a plumber is approximately $18 per hour. Apprentices usually earn half or $9 per hour

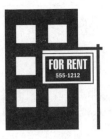

CHAPTER 2
RENTING AN APARTMENT

E veryone needs a place to live. How do you find an apartment? It is actually very easy if you are organized and know what to look for. But before you take that first cozy little studio or one bedroom bachelor pad that's within your budget, take a step back and consider what really matters about your "permanent" residence. Is it the location or neighborhood? Is it the size of the apartment? Or is it just the fabulous community pool? All are critical factors when choosing a place to live. So how can you possibly decide? Well, start by making a checklist of all the things that you want in an apartment such as the location, apartment size, and amenities (i.e., pool, balcony, parking). To help you develop such a list, Box 3 provides a checklist that you can use when looking at various apartments.

The important thing to remember is that there is more to selecting an apartment than just the size and price. Are the neighborhood, building, and common areas (parking, laundry, hallways) safe and secure? Are pets permitted? What about the laundry facilities? Are they in the unit, down the hall, or in the basement that is too dingy to even enter? What about the water pressure? Will it take you two hours to get the shampoo out of your hair under dribbling water?

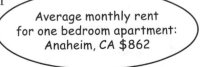

Average monthly rent for one bedroom apartment: Anaheim, CA $862

```
┌─────────────────────────────────────────────────────────┐
│                  BOX 3: APARTMENT FEATURES                │
│                                                           │
│                                         Example           │
│         General Apartment Information:                    │
│            Address                       123 Main St      │
│            Number of Bedrooms            1                │
│            Number of Bathrooms           1.5              │
│            Square Footage                925              │
│            Utilities Included            Gas              │
│            Monthly Rent                  $500             │
│            Money Due at Move-in          $800             │
│                                                           │
│         Apartment Features:                               │
│            Location (Basement, Top Floor, etc.)  Top      │
│            Central Air Conditioning      Yes              │
│            Bedroom Size                  Small            │
│            Closet Space                  Good             │
│            Flooring (Carpeting vs. Hardwood)  Carpet      │
│            Separate Dining Room/Area     No               │
│            Balcony/Deck                  Yes              │
│            Amount of Natural Light in Unit    Good        │
│            Fireplace                     No               │
│            Washer/Dryer in Unit          No               │
│            Refrigerator                  Yes              │
│            Dishwasher                     Yes             │
│            Built-In Microwave            Yes              │
│            Garbage Disposal              Yes              │
│                                                           │
│         Community/Building Features:                      │
│            Pets Allowed                  Yes              │
│            Parking                       Street           │
│            Laundry Facilities            Down hall        │
│            Pool/Recreation Facilities    Pool             │
│                                                           │
│         Neighborhood Features:                            │
│            Proximity to Work/School      Close            │
│            Proximity to Shopping Areas   Okay             │
│            Proximity to Recreation/Entertainment  Close   │
└─────────────────────────────────────────────────────────┘
```

What about natural light in the unit; do you want all your plants to die? Have you considered the amount of closet space in the apartment? These are just some of the items that are often overlooked by people that can make life difficult once you finally move into your place. By making a list of all the important factors before choosing a place, you will save yourself a lot of pain and anguish in the long run.

You've got your checklist so it's time to starting looking at apartments, right? Wrong! It's time to let your fingers do the walking, or rather, typing. There are a number of apartment search websites that include detailed descriptions allowing you to rank various apartments using your

> Average monthly rent for one bedroom apartment: Buffalo, NY $423

checklist without wasting time driving around and looking at each place. A simple web search can provide a list of apartments for rent and leasing companies in your area. If the website doesn't provide enough information, use that old-fashioned device called the telephone. Call and ask about the key items on your checklist. Use the list you've created to get as many questions answered *before* you actually begin looking at apartments so you will know what areas you need to address when you are meeting with various landlords.

Once you've identified apartments that meet your key needs and you have your checklist in hand, it's time for the fun part—looking at apartments! There is no magic number of apartments to view but you should look at several to make sure that you are getting the best place for your money. Don't forget that this is going to be your home for a while so it's okay to take your time and view numerous apartments before making your final decision. Make sure you are comfortable with the neighborhood and that it is safe. The main thing to remember when viewing apartments is not to be shy. Ask all the questions you want. Look in every room and in every closet.

> Average monthly rent for one bedroom apartment: Charlotte, NC $547

Turn on the shower. Notice where the phone jacks and electrical outlets are located. Ask about high-speed Internet connection availability.

Basically, just picture yourself going about your daily routine in the apartment. And take your time. You will likely get only one or maybe two opportunities to see the place before you have to make a decision. Also, if a copy of the floor plan with the room dimensions isn't available, have a tape measure with you and do your own measurements.

You do want your furniture to fit, don't you? Don't forget to measure the width of the doorway, hallway, and elevator. You can have the biggest

Average monthly rent for one bedroom apartment: Columbus, OH $472

apartment in the world but if your stuff won't fit through the door, it isn't coming in!

Make the apartment manager or landlord take you to all the common areas (i.e., pool, laundry facilities, parking garage). You are going to be spending a lot of your hard-earned money on rent so you don't want any unpleasant surprises after you move in. Plus, the demeanor of the apartment manager/landlord in response to your requests will give you some insight as to how dealing with this person will be when the inevitable issues arise (like fixing a clogged sink). After you leave, jot down a few notes on the place. Fill in any outstanding items on your apartment comparison worksheet that you couldn't get answered over the phone. This will help you evaluate apartments and come to your final decision.

Now that you have a couple of apartments that meet your requirements, you need to gather the paperwork the landlord will need in order to rent you the apartment. Although you can wait until after you have narrowed your search to one place, it is often a good idea to prepare this information before you even see any apartments. In some cities (e.g., New York), apartments are in such

Average monthly rent for one bedroom apartment: Milwaukee, WI $490

demand that they can be rented in only a few hours from the time they first become available. Wherever you live, you will need to pull together information on yourself, your job, your income, your finances, and any past landlords (see Box 4). Put all this information in one folder that you can take with

---

BOX 4: RENTAL APPLICATION MATERIALS

Current Employment Information:
  Name, Address and Phone Number of Employer
  Copy of Recent Paystub

Previous Residence Information (last three years):
  Addresses for Residences
  Names, Addresses, and Phone Numbers of Landlords

Financial Information:
  Social Security Number
  Bank Name and Account Numbers (checking and savings)
  Credit Card Numbers and Balances from Recent Statements

---

you as you look at different apartments. You certainly don't want to lose your dream place simply because the person who looked at it right after you had all her facts together and took the apartment on the spot while you were scrambling to gather your information! Just follow the Boy Scout motto, "Be Prepared."

What information do you need? Well, you should have a copy of a recent pay stub to verify your income, the name, address, and contact information of your employer, and the name and address of any former landlords. Apartment management companies will then verify your bank account information, credit card balances, and monthly car payment. They will use all this information to determine whether or not you can afford the apartment and if you have been a good tenant in the past.

Take a look at Box 5 to see how apartment managers often calculate whether a prospective tenant can afford the apartment. Notice that the national median of 27.2% of gross income spent on housing is within the suggested range of 25% to 30%. During this part of your search, you will likely be asked to write a non-refundable

Average monthly rent for one bedroom apartment: Dallas, TX $608 check for $20–$50 to cover the cost of running a credit report. This is standard practice when renting an apartment. Most management companies will then be able to let you know if you are approved to rent the apartment within a few days.

BOX 5: QUALIFYING FOR AN APARTMENT

		Example
Average Monthly Rent (1 Bedroom)*		$ 553
Months in a Year	×	12
Total Annual Rent		$ 6,636
Annual Rent as a % of Gross Income*	÷	27.2%
Income Necessary to Afford This Apartment		$ 24,397

*Based on National Median (Source: U.S. Census Bureau)

Congratulations! You've found a great apartment and have been approved. It's almost time to move in. But first, you've got to sign the paperwork and pay money (see Box 6). Most places will require a security deposit for any damage that you may do to the apartment during your occupancy. This can range from $100 to a full month's rent (or even two month's rent in some cases). Given that you already did your research when developing your checklist, this shouldn't come as any surprise. Ensure the amount requested for a security deposit is typical for your area and type of apartment. Ask what is considered "normal wear and tear" on your unit so that there won't be any disagreements when you move out. You do want to get your entire security deposit back, don't you? Also, even though you haven't even moved in, clarify what type of cleaning you will be expected to do upon moving out. Will the carpet have to be professionally cleaned or not? Additionally, some states require that the landlord pay interest on your security deposit. If this is the case, the interest rate should be specified in the paperwork.

Average monthly rent for one bedroom apartment: Kansas City, MO $506

In addition to the security deposit, you may need to pay your first month's (and maybe even your last month's) rent at this point. Be clear on the type of payment the landlord is expecting: personal check, certified check, or money order? Confirm when and where the rent payment is to be made. Is there any grace period? For example, many places require rent to be paid on the first of the month but will accept payments until the fifth of the month with no penalty.

Box 6: Money Due At Time Of Move

	Example
Security Deposit	$ 200
Pet Deposit*	$ 100
First Month's Rent	$ 500
Last Month's Rent*	$ 500
Total for Apartment	$ 1,300
Cable Company*	$ 50
Power Company*	$ 25
Phone Company*	$ 0
Other Utilities*	$ 0
Total for Utilities	$ 75
Total Due at Time of Move	$ 1,375

*may or may not be required

Ask about move-in/move-out fees. Some apartments require a separate security deposit for the elevator or charge a fee for you to move in or out. Are there any move-in restrictions or reservation requirements? There are apartment buildings that only allow one move-in per day. Since most moves occur around the beginning of the month, reserve the time slot you want. Imagine pulling up with a truck full of stuff only to be told you can't move into your new place because you didn't reserve the elevator!

Finally, when it comes time to sign the lease, read it first! Although this is not particularly enjoyable reading, you should take your time, read it completely, and ask any questions you may have. Don't just accept the landlord's assurances that, "It's a standard lease." It may be standard for the landlord since he does this for a living, but not for you. Remember, this is a legally binding contract. Be sure you are comfortable with everything in the lease before you sign it. Don't forget to get copies of all the paperwork after you are done signing everything.

Average monthly rent for one bedroom apartment: Portland, OR $559

Well, you now have a signed lease and are ready to move in. But there is one more thing you should do. What now?! Write down all the relevant landlord and maintenance staff contact information. In case there are any problems when you move in, you want to have this information handy in order to get any issues resolved quickly.

You've got a great new place and are ready to move in. Time to get your stuff packed and get into your new apartment already!

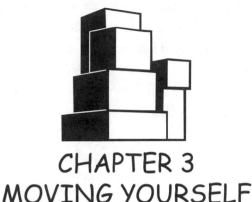

CHAPTER 3
MOVING YOURSELF

So it's time to move. Let's face it, moving is not fun. Whether you move yourself or even if you have the luxury of hiring professional movers, the process of moving can be a real pain. But don't despair. There are several things you can do and some tricks of the trade that can lessen the pain and simplify the process.

First, like many complex tasks, an old adage applies: "Plan your work then work your plan." Don't start the move by jamming everything you own into boxes in some haphazard way. Get completely organized before the first item goes into a box. It's often best to start by answering some questions and creating a checklist before springing into action.

How much stuff do you have? This is a generic, open-ended question that is tough to answer but it's the same one movers and truck rental companies will ask you right off the bat. What do they mean? Well, they're not really interested in specifically what you have—a big screen TV, a set of bunk beds, four bean bag chairs, and a collection of coffee mugs from all 50 states. Movers want to know how many "rooms" you have or the size of the apartment you'll be moving into.

About 43 million Americans move each year

Most people starting out will be moving into a one-bedroom apartment and therefore usually have two or three rooms. The bedroom is room one, the living room is room two, and the kitchen may or may not be room three. In a larger apartment, the kitchen may be big enough for a table or there may be a separate dining area, in either case, count this as room three. In a smaller apartment, the kitchen may be small and/or there is no separate dining area, so you'd want to think in terms of having only two full rooms.

One third of renters move every year

Whatever situation you find yourself in, there is no need to count the bathroom as a separate room. You certainly won't be bringing any furniture to your new bathroom and whatever towels and knick-knacks you have can easily be combined with one of the other rooms.

Finally, when determining how many rooms you have, consider the actual amount of furniture you'll be moving. Make a list of all the furniture you have. You'll need this information for the master packing list anyway, but it can be helpful now in determining how much stuff you have (see Box 7).

Bedroom furniture typically consists of a bed including mattress, box spring, frame and/or headboard along with a dresser, bureau, bedside tables, and lamps. Living room furniture includes a couch, chairs, coffee table, end tables, TV, stereo, entertainment center, and lamps. The kitchen/dining room has all the pots and pans, dishes, glasses, small kitchen appliances (microwave, coffeepot, blender, etc.) as well as a table and chairs. Other miscellaneous items to consider include extras like a desk, computer, file cabinets, TV for the bedroom, plants, framed pictures, art, sports equipment, and last but not least, clothes.

More than 3 million people move each year in order to establish their own household

Once you've made a list of all your stuff, tally it up. Again, think

BOX 7: SAMPLE MASTER PACKING LIST

	Packed	Delivered
Living Room		
Couch	√	√
Chairs	√	√
End Table	√	√
TV	√	√
Stereo	√	√
DVD/VCR	√	√
Lamps	√	√
Living Room Box 1: DVDs/CDs	√	√
Living Room Box 2: Books/Misc.	√	√
Kitchen/Dining Room		
Table	√	√
Chairs	√	√
Microwave	√	√
Coffee Maker	√	√
Kitchen Box 1: Pots and Pans	√	√
Kitchen Box 2: Plates and Glasses	√	√
Kitchen Box 3: Cleaning Supplies	√	√
Bedroom		
Mattress & Box Spring	√	√
Bed Frame/Headboard	√	√
Dresser	√	√
Bedside Table	√	√
Lamps	√	√
Bedroom Box 1: Wardrobe Box	√	√
Bedroom Box 2: Clothes	√	√
Bedroom Box 3: Clothes	√	√
Bedroom Box 4: Clothes	√	√
Bathroom		
Bathroom Box 1: Towels and Toiletries	√	√
Bathroom Box 2: Misc.	√	√
Miscellaneous		
Computer	√	√
File Cabinet	√	√
Sports Equipment	√	√

about the size of the new apartment. If you're in the larger apartment with the separate dining area but don't own a table and chairs, don't yet own a couch, and only have a twin bed, well, then you really have two rooms, not three.

If your new place is on the cozy side but you've got every piece of furniture listed above and are a clotheshorse, think of yourself as having three rooms. Don't forget that you've got to fit all this stuff in the new place and then live there. Consider getting rid of some stuff.

More people move out of the Northeast than anywhere else

Moving is a great time to do a little "spring cleaning" and toss some of your old clothes and other items before lugging all of it to your new place.

For the vast majority of people, hiring professional movers is too expensive. You'll have to schlep all of your belongings yourself together with a couple of friends you've conned into helping you by promising them pizza and beer, or worse, by agreeing to help them when they move. At this point, all you've determined is how much stuff you have. Now you have to rent a truck to move everything. Two common sizes are the 14-foot and the 10-foot truck. Remember, the smaller truck will drive more like a pick-up, will more likely have automatic instead of stick-shift transmission, and will be easier to maneuver and park (and don't forget about air conditioning for a long summer drive). On the flip side, the larger truck may be easier to pack and fit everything inside.

Time to let your fingers do the walking and dial around to various truck rental companies. Start with the Big Boys: Uhaul, Ryder, Budget, and Penske. These companies can often be the best for a one-way move from one city to another since they are nationwide and can offer the best rates. These companies can also be your best option for a local move where you pick up the truck in the morning and

The most popular moving destination is the South

return it back to the same location at the end of the day. Consider where you have to pick up and return the truck as part of your decision in which company to choose if price is similar. There are also local or regional companies that are great for cross-town moves or short moves less than 50 miles. Don't forget to call these companies.

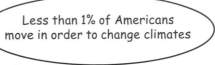

Less than 1% of Americans move in order to change climates

When you call around to the various truck renters, remember to ask a few specifics. Confirm the availability of your particular truck (e.g. a 10-footer), the exact time you can pick it up on moving day (say 8 a.m.), when the truck is due back (say 7 p.m.), and exactly where to return the truck. If the company is still open when you return the truck, returning it is easy enough. But often the rental office closes long before you'll be done with the truck in which case you'll be returning the truck "after hours." This is standard in the industry. For example, the office may close at 5 p.m. but as long as the truck is returned before seven the next morning, you won't be charged for an extra day. But you'll need to know the procedure as to where to park the truck and what to do with the keys when you go to return it at 8 p.m.

Finally, most rental companies record any existing damage to the truck when you pick it up (and all of these trucks seem to have a few scrapes and dings). Note whatever damage the truck already has so that you are not charged for any pre-existing dents when you return the vehicle.

Approximately 1/3 of all 20-29-year-olds move each year

Most truck rental companies also have moving supplies available for both purchase and rent. Stock up on these items to make your move as painless as possible. The most needed are cardboard boxes and packing tape. Boxes are shockingly expensive so if you can get your hands on any used ones floating around in decent condition, grab 'em. You'll have to splurge for the packing tape because regular tape doesn't hold up so well and you want to be sure your boxes don't fall apart during transit or while carrying them up three flights of stairs. Even if you get a hold of some used boxes, you'll likely have to purchase some new ones as well. Buy all your moving supplies in advance of the move. Remember, you really want to pack everything before you move and not wait until after you've already picked up the truck. Packing your boxes and furniture well in advance will make your move go much more smoothly.

1 in 3 Americans rent rather than own their housing

Consider buying one or two specialty boxes such as a wardrobe box. This baby acts as a movable closet complete with a metal hanging bar across the top. Your entire closet can be dropped right into the wardrobe box with shirts and pants still on the hangers. It couldn't be simpler and is well worth the investment.

Another item available for rent is a dolly or hand truck. It is usually only $5 or $10 for the day and is a lifesaver (and back saver) for moving heavy items and also for moving stacks of boxes at once instead of one at a time. If you're moving any appliances such as a refrigerator or washer and dryer, you'll almost certainly be renting a hand truck.

Blankets and padding are another wise rental investment. For only a few bucks you'll be able to wrap up all your fragile or bulky items, just like professional movers, and not worry about breakage or dents. Blankets are especially great for wrapping up your TV.

Okay, it's a couple days before the big move, time to actually box up all your stuff. Let's review a few packing tips (see Box 8).

There are nearly 36 million renter-occupied housing units in the U.S.

First, to the extent you can, pack by room. It doesn't make sense to pack pillowcases in the same box with a frying pan, your stereo, and bath towels. By packing by room,

---

Box 8: Packing Tips

- Organize what you have to pack before you start packing
- Make a list of all of your furniture and large items
- Do some "spring cleaning" (i.e., get rid of some stuff)
- Write down the details of renting a truck
- Buy all of your moving supplies (e.g., boxes) in advance
- Consider buying some specialty boxes (e.g., a wardrobe box)
- Rent a dolly or hand truck
- Grab a couple old blankets for wrapping furniture
- Pack by room
- Label each box with a number and contents on the front, left-hand corner
- Record each box and furniture item on your master packing list
- Put the boxes in the appropriate room at your new place to make unpacking easier

---

it's easier to catalog all items on the master packing list, keep track of items during the packing phase, put each box in the proper room of the new place, and simplify the unpacking process.

In addition to cataloging the items on the master packing list, label each box on the outside (a magic marker or Sharpie is best) by room and content, "Bedroom: Clothes (Box 1 of 4)." Don't label on the top of the box since you won't be able to read it when you stack boxes, be consistent and use the upper left-hand corner of the front side of the box instead.

When filling your boxes, be aware of the weight of the items. It's not a good idea to overload boxes with heavy items. Boxes can tear apart, are difficult and awkward to carry, and put unnecessary strain on your back. Fill up the bottom half of a box with heavier items but then place lighter items on top.

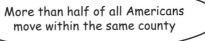

More than half of all Americans move within the same county

Books are a perfect example of heavier items that should be spread around to several boxes. This also helps to stabilize the boxes when stacking them three or four high. When packing fragile items, use towels, T-shirts, and blankets to cover the items to provide cushion. Wrap kitchen items such as dishes and glassware in old newspaper; it's free and is still the best way to keep things from breaking.

Finally, what to do with odd-size and other loose items? Box them up. Go ahead and pack things like the telephone, remote controls, sports equipment, and other small items. A lot of this stuff is easy enough to carry unboxed and may seem like a waste of box space, but remember, each item requires another trip up and down the stairs and everything has to go in the truck. It is much easier to pack the truck with four extra boxes than with half a dozen lose items bouncing around. Plus, if you've rented the hand truck, you can wheel these boxed items around in one fell swoop.

Now for the most important packing tip: less is more. The less you actually have to pack, the easier your move will be. Moving is a great time to clean out your closet and eliminate unwanted and unused gear. Take the time to do this before you move. Why box it up, carry it across town, move it into your new place, unpack it, and then decide that you haven't worn it in three years and don't want it anymore? The same goes for furniture. If you're not going to use it, or plan on replacing it within a couple of weeks of moving, get rid of it now.

About 60% of Americans live in the state in which they were born

The Salvation Army, Goodwill, Volunteers of America, and even your local church, in addition to taking old clothes, may accept donations of furniture, small appliances, and sports equipment. Plus, in many cities, these organizations will come to your place and pick the items up and haul them away. When calling these organizations, have a list of the items you wish to donate ready. Don't forget to get a receipt for any items you give away for tax purposes. Donating clothing and furniture simplifies your move, is a tax-deductible endeavor, and helps out those less fortunate in your local community.

If you still have too much stuff but don't want to give it away, consider renting a storage unit. They are perfect for storing large items or furniture that you know you want down the road but don't have room for in your new apartment. Public storage units are quite affordable and available practically everywhere. Of course, the greatest (and cheapest) "storage unit" is still your parents' attic or a friend's basement!

It's moving day. Everything is packed and ready, you've picked up the truck, and now it's time to actually load the truck. Intimidating. Start big and heavy and move to small and light. Typically your couch, mattress/box spring, and a dresser are the biggest (and bulkiest) items. Put the mattress and box spring on their sides and lean them up against one of the walls of the truck. Use the couch to hold the bed upright in place. Turn the couch so the front is against the mattress to create a "pocket" between the mattress and the back of the couch. A number of boxes and other items will fit nicely in here and will be wedged in so nothing can slide around.

Other large and heavy pieces of furniture can fit all the way forward in the truck and down the side opposite the bed and couch. Also, lining the bed of the truck with a blanket allows you to lay a table upside down (with table legs sticking up in the air). You can then stack boxes 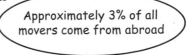 and other items on the inverted table to secure it in place and not take up any space in the truck. Get as many of the larger items into the truck as soon as you can as it is much easier to tuck boxes and smaller items in and around the big pieces. Blankets come in handy to cushion larger items. Remember that all of the items will shift and slide during transit so position items securely.

That's it—the truck is all packed and it's off to your new place!

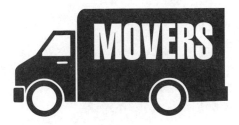

CHAPTER 4
HIRING PROFESSIONAL MOVERS

S ay you're lucky enough to be able to afford professional movers. How do you decide whom to use? If you open the Yellow Pages to "Movers" the sheer number of choices will blow you away. Well, with something like moving, there is no better selection guide than word-of-mouth and personal recommendation. Ask around.

Do you have any friends who moved recently? What about anyone at your job? Talk to them. Who did they use? How much did it cost? Where there any hidden costs? Did the movers show up on time? Did the movers break anything? Did they wrap furniture with blankets and pads before moving? What about at the end of the day, how much did the person tip the mover? Basically, whatever contacts you have, be sure to pump them for as much information as possible. Even if the person had a horrible moving experience, it's still valuable information—take that company off your list.

Among the dozens of companies from which to choose, if you find a company that one or two friends have used successfully, hire that company. If it ain't broke, don't fix it. You can still price shop a bit by calling around, but in the end, like with most things, in moving you get what you pay for. These are all of your worldly possessions they're

> 1 in 6 Americans moves for work-related reasons

moving. Spending an extra $50 to hire a company that someone you know has used before and recommended can be some of the best money ever spent.

Another thought when using professional movers: insurance. Be sure to ask about the standard insurance included in the price quoted

From 1995-2000, nearly half of the U.S. population over age 5 moved

for the move as well as the cost of additional insurance. Understand the difference between "damage value" and "replacement value." Your TV may only be worth $200 since it's a few years old, but if the movers drop it, are you entitled to the $200 damage value of the item or the $500 replacement value it would cost to buy a brand new TV? Buying additional insurance may seem like throwing money away but could seem like a bargain should your stuff end up strewn across the highway after a collision with a manure spreader on the Santa Ana Freeway.

There are a number of items to address when selecting a professional mover (see Box 9). Confirm how the movers charge: flat rate, by mileage/distance, by the hour (usually with a minimum), or some combination, i.e. $50 per hour plus $0.30 per mile for each mile greater than 25 miles. If the company does charge by the hour, ask how many movers they will be sending to do your move. Obviously, three guys can move faster than only two movers.

Regardless of how they charge, be sure to get a pre-move quote or estimate. You've already pulled together all the information a moving company will need in order to estimate the cost of the move so be sure to get a quote. If they can't or won't provide you with an estimate, you may want to consider choosing a different mover.

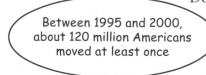

Between 1995 and 2000, about 120 million Americans moved at least once

Don't let the person on the phone hem and haw about how every move is different, they can't tell how long it will take until they get there, it depends on how much stuff you have, how's it's packed, etc. These guys are professional movers and supposedly have been moving people for years. If they aren't comfortable giving you a ballpark figure, do you really want to put your possessions in their hands?

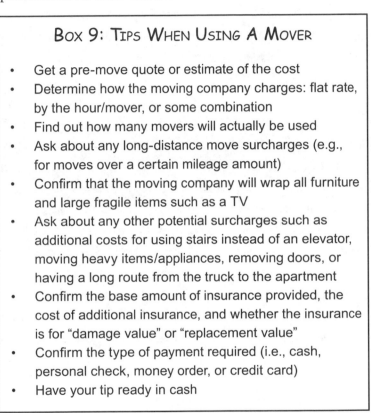

BOX 9: TIPS WHEN USING A MOVER

- Get a pre-move quote or estimate of the cost
- Determine how the moving company charges: flat rate, by the hour/mover, or some combination
- Find out how many movers will actually be used
- Ask about any long-distance move surcharges (e.g., for moves over a certain mileage amount)
- Confirm that the moving company will wrap all furniture and large fragile items such as a TV
- Ask about any other potential surcharges such as additional costs for using stairs instead of an elevator, moving heavy items/appliances, removing doors, or having a long route from the truck to the apartment
- Confirm the base amount of insurance provided, the cost of additional insurance, and whether the insurance is for "damage value" or "replacement value"
- Confirm the type of payment required (i.e., cash, personal check, money order, or credit card)
- Have your tip ready in cash

That said, even the most experienced and reliable movers won't be able to give you a quote down to the penny. Every move is different. But by getting an estimate up front, you'll know approximately what it will cost and are protected from getting hit with a wildly higher figure at the end of the move.

There are a few other things that can run up the cost of the actual move so you should ask about these items ahead of time. What are these potential "hidden" charges? Well, movers often have surcharges for things like using stairs instead of an elevator,

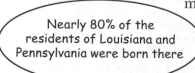

Nearly 80% of the residents of Louisiana and Pennsylvania were born there

moving a particularly heavy piece of furniture, removing doors from their hinges to squeeze a couch through a tight doorway (which won't happen to you since you measured the doorways when you looked for the apartment!), or carrying all of the stuff a particularly long distance from the truck to the apartment. By asking about all of these items up front when you book the movers, you'll have no surprises on moving day.

When the movers arrive at your place to start the move, be prepared. Have all your stuff ready to go and your master packing list all filled out (Box 7). There's nothing more frustrating for professional movers than to show up at someone's apartment only to discover that the person is only half-packed. Plus, don't forget that the longer the movers have to wait around for you to get your stuff ready, the more expensive your move will be. Time is money.

A final piece of advice when using professional movers—treat them with respect. Even though they are working for you, don't order them around like servants. Aside from the fact that being courteous is the right thing to do, don't forget that these guys are handling all of your worldly goods! Offer them a glass of water or cold drink during the move.

Finally, once everything is moved in and all the paperwork is completed, give them a tip in cash. A good guideline to start with is between 15% and 20% of the total cost just like in a restaurant. The tip should be at least $20 per person and perhaps as much as $40 each. There is usually one guy in charge so you can give the entire tip to him and let him split it up among the crew.

Only 21% of the residents of Nevada were born there

You're done. Your wallet may be a bit lighter, but at least by using professional movers, your back isn't sore!

CHAPTER 5
SETTLING IN

Now you're all moved in! You and your friends (or your wallet) are exhausted from moving all your stuff. You're finished right? Well, not quite. Aside from the fact that you still have to unpack everything, there are a few loose ends to tie.

Did you remember to fill out a change of address form with the post office? You can actually do this several weeks in advance and the post office will begin forwarding your mail the day you move into the new apartment (and will continue to forward your mail for six months).

You'll need to change your address with every company and organization with which you correspond. These include your bank, credit card companies, magazine subscriptions, employer, health insurance provider, clubs, and of course, friends and family. One way to make your life easy is to change your address with the post office first. Then, as you receive each piece of mail or bill that's been forwarded to your new address, you can update each company with the new address whenever you pay the bill or get mail from them.

Now everyone knows where to find you. Your mail is on its way. Kick back, relax, turn on the A/C, cook up some

> 71% of households with income between $15,000 and $30,000 have cable or satellite TV

dinner, flip on the tube, log on to your e-mail, and call a friend. Oh wait. You have no A/C because you have no power. The stove has no gas. The TV is all snow since you have no cable. Ditto for the cable modem for your high speed Internet connection. And you have no dial tone when you plug in the phone. You forgot to

> Nearly half the U.S. population uses e-mail

get the utilities hooked up! Most people wait until they've moved in to discover/remember to do this. Why? Just like changing your address with the post office, you can make arrangements to have utilities turned on and schedule appointments before you move.

Basic utilities such as electricity, gas, and water (if not included in your rent) can all be turned on by the providers the day you move in. Calling them in advance will ensure that they "flip the switch" first thing the morning of your moving day. This is critical on a hot summer day to have the A/C going, cold drinks in the fridge, and the ability to use the bathroom. If you've had these utilities in your name at another address in the same service area, the utility companies can usually turn on your service without you having to do anything other than call them. If not, depending on the provider and state laws, you may have to fill out certain paperwork in advance or provide a small security deposit before they will hook up the utilities (this is not uncommon for first-time renters). By calling a few weeks in advance, you'll be able ensure that all your ducks are in a row on moving day. When you rented the apartment, the landlord should have provided you with the utility information and phone numbers for exactly this purpose. If not, Box 10 is an example of how to organize your utility

> 2 out of 3 Americans use a computer at home, work, or school

company information.

The same may hold true for other non-basic (but perhaps more important) utilities such as telephone, cable, satellite, and high speed Internet (DSL or cable modem). Again, if you've been a previous subscriber you may not have to do anything other than call. But you may be required to fill out paperwork and/or provide a security deposit. Regardless, sometimes the company can flip a switch, other times you may need to schedule an appointment for a technician to come out to your apartment. If you get lucky and the tenant before you already had things set up for the phone, cable,

---

Box 10: Move-In Service Checklist

Company	Phone	Called For Service
Phone	555-XXXX	√
Cable	555-XXXX	√
Satellite	555-XXXX	√
Internet	555-XXXX	√
Gas	555-XXXX	√
Water	555-XXXX	√
Electric	555-XXXX	√

---

and Internet, an appointment may not be necessary. By calling a couple weeks in advance, you can be sure that if an appointment is necessary, you'll have it scheduled for the day after you move in.

It's pretty chaotic on moving day so it is strongly advised that you not schedule the cable guy to show up in the middle of your move. Go without cable for a day and have the technician show up the next morning. If you're a careful planner, it is possible to have the installer show up first thing in the morning before you've even shown up with your truckload of goods. But remember

> From 1998 to 2001, Internet access doubled from approximately 25% to over 50% of all households in America

that someone has to be there to let him in, sign the paperwork, and pay whatever installation fee is due. Cable access usually requires the installation fee and first month's usage fee to be paid directly to the technician, sometimes in cash. Confirm this with the utility company when scheduling the appointment.

One final tip. If you've moved yourself, you've rented a truck for the day. Depending on the size of your move, how far you're moving, and how many people you've roped into helping, you could finish unloading everything by mid-afternoon. Don't be in a hurry to immediately return the truck. It's already paid for, is there anyway else you can use it? One great idea is to determine before you move if there are any new items or furniture you'll need for the new apartment. If you need a table and chairs, a new couch, mattress, or any other large or bulky items, go shopping a week or so before the move. Many stores have delivery charges of $25 to $100 or more for these pieces of furniture. Save yourself this money by picking up your new stuff in your now-empty rental truck.

Even if you aren't buying new furniture, the truck could still be useful. A trip to Wal-Mart, Home Depot, or a similar store might be necessary to buy odds-and-

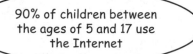

90% of children between the ages of 5 and 17 use the Internet

ends and bulky items. Things like outdoor garbage cans, indoor trash cans, brooms or mops, potted plants or flowers, or anything that might not easily fit into your car or would dirty the back seat is the perfect item to throw in the back of the rental truck. Make sure you've gotten the full value out of the truck before you return it.

Congratulations! Now you really are moved in. Well, your stuff is all moved. Bed is unassembled, furniture is jammed in a corner of the living room, boxes are strewn about the entire apartment, and good luck finding whatever article of clothing you suddenly need at the moment. You're moved, just not unpacked. This is about the time when your friends demand the pizza and beer, eat and drink it, and then disappear. It's up to you to put everything away and focus on making your apartment into a place you can call home.

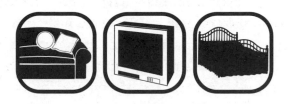

CHAPTER 6
FURNISHING YOUR HOME: THE BIG STUFF

With all the boxes unpacked and the furniture in place, it's time to take a look around. Is your new apartment a *house* or is it a *home*? In other words, does it feel like the place you're comfortable calling home for at least the next year or is it simply four bare walls with scattered furniture and a place to crash? Well, regardless of your budget there are several things you can do to make yourself feel more comfortable and get settled in as soon as possible.

No matter where you've been living, you're going to need some things to furnish your new place. This is especially true if you were living at home or if you had a roommate; some of the furniture and other household items belonged to them and not you. Even if you are moving in with a roommate now, there will still be items you'll want to buy. What are they?

Let's start by taking a quick inventory of the major furniture in most apartments. Not every apartment will have all of these items, some will have more, some will have less, but it's an excellent way to start. Let's go room by room.

> 29% of households with income between $15,000 and $30,000 have a large screen TV

Your basic living room has a couch, a coffee table, and a TV on some sort of stand. Existing without these three items is not much fun. It's nice if the room has another chair, an end table, a lamp, and maybe an entertainment center that can also house a stereo, VCR, or DVD player. You don't have to have all of this, but if you do, you're pretty much set.

12% of households with income between $15,000 and $30,000 have two or more refrigerators

In the bedroom, all you really need is a bed, a dresser or chest of drawers of some sort, and maybe a bedside table and lamp. That's really it. It's nice to get all kinds of other items and matching sets but it certainly isn't necessary when starting out. You need a place to sleep, to store your socks, T-shirts, and unmentionables, and to keep an alarm clock. Everything else goes in the closet.

If your apartment has a dining area or a large kitchen, it's great to have a table and chairs. Every once in a while it's nice to eat a meal while actually seated at a table instead of hunched over the coffee table while watching TV. This is especially true if you ever cook dinner for a date or if your parents insist on stopping by. A dining room table isn't just for dining as it also makes a great workspace to go through the mail, pay bills, and set up a desktop or laptop computer if you don't have a separate desk area.

Okay, so that's all the furniture you need to really set yourself up in your new place. Don't worry if you don't have every piece of furniture you want when you first move into your place; you can pick them up in the coming months as your budget allows. This apartment is your place so you can furnish it however you wish. That's the beauty of living on your own—no one to tell you how to do things or what to have in your apartment. If you find yourself at the opposite end of the

40% of households with income between $15,000 and $30,000 have a dishwasher

spectrum and have every conceivable piece of furniture and home furnishing item, that's okay too. If everything fits in the apartment without overwhelming the place, that's terrific.

But let's assume that you do need a few of the items. There are a few tips that can allow you to furnish your place in style without breaking the bank (see Box 11). An obvious statement is that if you need furniture, go to a furniture store. Well, that's true but they can

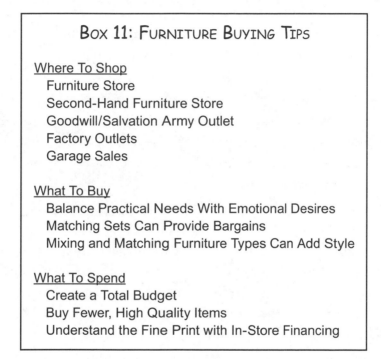

Box 11: Furniture Buying Tips

<u>Where To Shop</u>
  Furniture Store
  Second-Hand Furniture Store
  Goodwill/Salvation Army Outlet
  Factory Outlets
  Garage Sales

<u>What To Buy</u>
  Balance Practical Needs With Emotional Desires
  Matching Sets Can Provide Bargains
  Mixing and Matching Furniture Types Can Add Style

<u>What To Spend</u>
  Create a Total Budget
  Buy Fewer, High Quality Items
  Understand the Fine Print with In-Store Financing

be expensive. Make sure to look in the paper and keep your eyes open for sales at the major furniture stores. Sale weekends (e.g., Memorial Day or Labor Day) are often great opportunities to pick up new furniture at a substantial discount.

An item to pay close attention to when buying items at a furniture store is the in-store financing. While many stores offer great deals and allow you to pay for the items much later, be sure to read the fine print. The due date for your full payment is critical. If you pay by that time, the interest charges may be waived. But often, if you miss the date or don't pay the entire amount at that point, the interest will not be waived and you may then owe both the original price plus the interest that built up since you purchased the items. As you consider using the in-store financing option, make sure you understand exactly how much is due and when it is due.

Also, try going to a second-hand furniture store where you can get great stuff that may be slightly used or worn but at a fraction of the cost of new furniture. Remember when you donated that old and terribly ugly couch to Goodwill or the Salvation Army before you moved into your new place? Well, these organizations collect and refurbish other people's items as well. Don't forget the old adage, "One man's trash is another man's treasure." If one of these organizations has a household goods outlet (as opposed to merely used clothing) in your town, you have an excellent chance of picking up quality items at a deep discount.

65% of households with income between $15,000 and $30,000 have a washer and dryer

Finally, nothing beats a good, old-fashioned garage sale. Even in the Internet age and the advent of online auctions, perusing the newspaper for weekend yard sale announcements is often the best way to go. Face it, you can't ship a used couch through the mail. And there is no better way to determine if you like the color or if it's comfortable than to see it in person and plop down on it. Plus, like everything at a garage sale, the price is negotiable.

When out bargain-hunting for new furniture and odds-and-ends, you definitely want to have a budget and keep in mind how one particular item's price may impact what you can pay for other items. If you only have $300 to spend but need half a dozen things, it may not be best to blow $250 on a dresser or the rest of the items you buy may end up being glorified junk.

Another critical factor to remember—quality counts. You could end up owning many of the items of furniture you purchase for a lot longer than you think. It happens all the time. A person is deciding between two couches: one she doesn't really like for $150 and another she likes a lot better but costs $250. She decides to save $100 and get the cheaper couch because even though she doesn't really like it, it makes no difference since she plans on buying a brand new couch in six months when she has more money. Five years later, she still has that god-awful, ugly $150 couch that she absolutely hates. Not only that, she's moved the hideous thing to three different apartments over the years. Big items such as couches tend to stay with people much longer than anticipated. Don't break the bank, but buy something that doesn't turn your stomach.

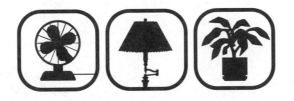

CHAPTER 7
FURNISHING YOUR HOME:
THE SMALL STUFF

Just because you have all the right furniture doesn't mean you are done furnishing your place. There is one room in the apartment that's been largely ignored to this point, the kitchen. Except for possibly a table, there really isn't any furniture but there are still many things needed in order to properly stock the kitchen. The basic items are dishes, glasses, silverware, pots and pans, and a few small pieces. Small appliances such as microwaves, blenders, toasters, and coffee makers are a matter of personal taste, but there is no getting around the need for the basics. There are three things to keep in mind when purchasing these items.

First, actually purchase them. Don't settle for your existing hodgepodge of mismatched, hand-me-down plates, bowls and glasses you've accumulated from Mom or by purchasing enough value meals to receive the special edition collector set. And plastic cups saved from sporting events don't cut it either. You'll be glad you have two plates the same size, shape, and color as one another should you ever have anyone over for dinner.

Second, less is more. When you're at the local Wal-Mart or discount store buying dishes and

> Approximately 13% of monthly expenditures are spent on food in the typical American household

glasses, don't get sucked in by the "Super-Duper Kitchen Starter Set Value Pack." You may get a big bang for your buck buying one of these, but do you really need a 48-piece glassware set of every conceivable shape and size? Maybe the house you grew up in had a unique glass for every type of beverage or had

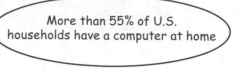

More than 55% of U.S. households have a computer at home

service for 16 people, but that's not what you need in your new place. You are only one person. A set of four is plenty. This goes for plates, bowls, glasses, and silverware. You'll spend less money, only have to do dishes once every four days, and still be able to offer three guests a beverage in a clean glass.

Third, once again, less is more. Quantity was just addressed, now let's talk about quality. Since you're only buying four plates and glasses, you may think you should buy high quality. Wrong! Glasses break all the time. You can get a set of four matching glasses for less than five dollars. That way, once you break them, it's only another five bucks and you're right back in business. The same goes for plates and silverware. Stuff gets chipped and broken on occasion. Don't kid yourself. You're not entertaining royalty in your place so no one expects fine china and polished silver. The fact that everything matches and doesn't contain a sports logo is good enough. Unlike your couch, which you could have for years, kitchen items are replaced regularly.

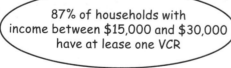

87% of households with income between $15,000 and $30,000 have at lease one VCR

A couple of other small items are needed for the kitchen even if you're not a gourmet chef. You may not plan on cooking very often or it may be a daily event, in either case, you will likely cook or heat up something at some point. At a minimum, you need one pot and one pan. The standard three-quart saucepan with a lid is a must. With it you can make soup, boil water to cook pasta, and basically heat up whatever liquids you need to. You also need either a seven-inch or ten-inch frying pan; it doesn't really matter. The frying pan is key to cooking eggs, making a grilled cheese sandwich, frying a burger, whatever. Any other pots and pans you can get your hands on are a bonus, but you need these two. When buying them, there is no need to spend a lot of money, perhaps no more than $20.

A couple of other utensils round out what you need to stock the most basic of kitchens. All of these items are cheap and there is no need to spend any more on each item than you have to. A colander for draining pasta, a pitcher for cold water, a wooden spoon, a plastic spatula for flipping burgers or frying eggs, a rubber spatula for scraping, a cookie/baking sheet for frozen pizzas, a wine corkscrew and one really good, sharp knife and cutting board. Box 12 provides a list of basic kitchen items to get you started.

Now let's talk very briefly about items for the bathroom as there is almost nothing to say. The only items you really need, beyond the requisite bathroom necessities, are towels and wash cloths. Same logic applies here as in the kitchen. Buy a cheap set of four and call it a day. Just the fact that the towels are all the same color and were not stolen from a motel or meant for the beach will dramatically improve the look of your bathroom. Plus, with a set of four, laundry can be postponed considerably and should you have an overnight

BOX 12: BASIC KITCHEN ITEMS	
Dishes –	Set of 4
Glasses –	Set of 4
Silverware –	Set of 4
Pots –	3-Quart Saucepan with Lid
Pans –	7" or 10" Frying Pan
Pitcher –	2-Quart
Utensils –	One Sharp Cutting Knife Cutting Board Colander Cookie/Baking Sheet Wooden Spoon Plastic Spatula Rubber Spatula Wine Corkscrew

guest, you'll be glad to be able to
give the person a clean towel
and not embarrass yourself
by handing him the one you
just used to dry off.

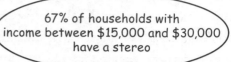

67% of households with
income between $15,000 and $30,000
have a stereo

Enough about the bathroom, let's go back to the kitchen. You have all the supplies, so what are you missing? Food! You still need to stock the cupboards and the fridge. It's not like you don't know what you like to eat and how to buy food at the grocery store, but there are a few useful tips and several money-saving suggestions to help you stock your kitchen for the first time.

First, where to shop? In order to save money, people are quick to sing the praises of the various warehouse clubs, discount stores, and volume purchase outlets. In many homes, perhaps yours growing up, these stores were the only place to shop for the family's groceries. True, these places offer terrific savings when buying multiple items in bulk or large quantities of a single item. That's why they are so perfect for families. But are they right for you now that you're on your own? Maybe. Only you know your shopping and eating habits. However, they aren't the only paths to savings particularly if you know you'll never finish a five-gallon drum of ice cream or a 40-lb. bag of rice. And don't forget that many of these warehouse clubs have a membership fee to

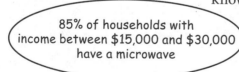

85% of households with
income between $15,000 and $30,000
have a microwave

join, perhaps as much as $50. You'll still save money in the long run, but maybe you can't afford the up-front costs.

There are alternatives. Nearly all grocery store chains and many independent, local stores have their own version of discount clubs. You've probably seen them in the store where you shop. A box of cereal is $2.79 but only $2.29 if you're a "member" of that store's discount club. How do you become a member? It's easy, all you have to do is sign up at the main cashier or office at the front of the store.

These in-store clubs are almost always free. You sign up, they give you a card for your wallet or key chain and before you check out, you just hand the card to the cashier and the price is automatically reduced as the cashier scans each item.

This type of club is perfect for a person living alone or with a roommate because the savings applies to each individual can of soup or jar of mayonnaise and doesn't require bulk purchasing. Many of these stores also offer a one-time discount of 5% or 10% on the entire purchase the day you sign up for the card. Be sure to ask about this because the day you go to the grocery store to stock up your new apartment for the first time can be one of the larger purchases you'll make.

55% of single person households eat at least one home-cooked, hot meal per day

So what do you need to buy? Again, everyone knows the staples and the foods they like but there are a few items to purchase on the first trip to stick in the cupboard for a rainy day and the daily items that are easily overlooked. Even if cooking isn't your thing, everyone needs a few spices and condiments. Start off with salt and pepper, oregano, and perhaps one all-purpose seasoning. A bottle of corn or olive oil and a bag of sugar (especially for coffee) are worth having around. Also, buy a few cans of soup and some pasta and sauce. This is in addition to whatever you might eat on a regular basis.

These "emergency" foods are perfect for a day when you're tired and hungry, open the fridge, and realize you have nothing at all to eat. You'll be thrilled when you check the cupboard and realize you can save yourself from running to the store by dipping into this emergency stash. Microwave popcorn is also the perfect food should you find yourself in this situation late at night. Finally, beyond the standard milk and bread, stock up on a few basic condiments for the fridge such

56% of households with income between $15,000 and $30,000 have an electric coffee maker

as butter, ketchup, mustard, mayonnaise, salsa, and salad dressing. Nothing is worse than making a sandwich only to discover you've got nothing to put on it!

Almost done. While at the store, throw a few bathroom and general cleaning supplies into the cart as well. Grab a bottle of all-purpose cleaner (e.g., Fantastic), glass cleaner (e.g., Windex), tub and tile cleaner (e.g., Soft Scrub), a generic cleanser or toilet bowl cleaner, and disinfectant (e.g., Lysol). Don't forget automatic dishwasher soap, regular dish soap, and laundry detergent as well. Throw in a sponge, mop, broom, dish towels, and possibly a vacuum cleaner and your new apartment will remain as spic-and-span as the day you moved in (see Box 13).

That's just about everything you need to know to turn your house into your home. You've stocked the kitchen cabinets, the cupboard, the fridge, and have everything you need to keep the place sparkling. But there are a few final tips to give your apartment the finishing touches to warm the place up and make it more inviting.

Box 13: Pantry Items

Spices/Condiments:
- Salt
- Pepper
- Oregano
- All-Purpose Seasoning
- Sugar
- Vegetable Oil
- Ketchup
- Mustard
- Mayonnaise
- Salsa
- Salad Dressing

Cleaning Supplies:
- Sponge
- Mop
- Broom
- Dish Towels
- Vacuum Cleaner
- Toilet Brush
- All-Purpose Cleaner
- Glass Cleaner
- Tub and Tile Cleaner
- Toilet Bowl Cleaner
- Disinfectant
- Dishwasher Soap
- Dish Soap
- Laundry Detergent

House plants are one of the cheapest ways to fill up blank walls or open areas, brighten up a room, and provide a warmer atmosphere. A half-dozen plants spread around an apartment can make an amazing and immediate change to the feel of your place. Don't worry if you don't have a green thumb, there are many varieties of plants that require a minimum of direct sunlight and water. At the store, read the card attached to the plant or ask a sales attendant.

If your new place is nothing more than a couch, coffee table, TV, and four blank walls, don't despair. Hanging a few framed photographs or posters will do the trick. Intimidated by the thought of hanging a picture or a series of pictures on a single wall? Cut pieces of paper the same size as the picture frames and then tape the paper to the wall where you want the picture to hang. You can easily tape and re-tape the paper to the wall as many times as you need to align photos or create the look you want. Once this is done, pound the nail right through the paper into the wall. Tear away the paper and hang your frames; it's that simple!

Approximately 65%-70% of residents in Alaska and Minnesota use the Internet, the highest usage rate in the nation

If you've got bare windows or an unsightly view, hanging some cheap curtains is often a great solution. Even if the windows came with pre-installed blinds, sometimes hanging a little fabric at the edges of the window is a great way to improve a room, soften a window, or disguise an unattractive view. Placing a plant or a few candles on the windowsill is another nice enhancement. Candles are also an inexpensive way to add color to a room and lighting a few in the evenings can create a warm and inviting atmosphere. All of these tips are inexpensive ways to get you feeling at home in your new apartment as quickly as possible.

Approximately 40%-45% of residents of Louisiana and Mississippi use the Internet, the lowest usage rate in the nation

That's got to be it, right? Just about. Now that you have all this great stuff in your apartment, you want to protect it don't you? That means renter's insurance. Many people neglect this insurance but what happens in the unlikely event of a break-in, flood, or fire?

Assuming that everyone in the apartment is okay, what about all your stuff? Can you really afford to furnish your apartment all over again? Renter's insurance is a relatively inexpensive way to protect your belongings in the case of some unforeseen event. Call around to different homeowner's insurance companies to get an estimate on how much this will cost.

Even if you don't think you have much of value to insure, do a quick tally of your possessions. With your couch, TV, stereo, CD collection, and computer you could have over $3,000 of valuable items. And don't forget about your clothes. Spending an extra $20 per month on renter's insurance could prove extraordinarily valuable in the long run. Plus, renter's insurance often covers other items used away from your apartment such as a mountain bike or a laptop computer. You have insurance to cover yourself and your car, so don't forget to get insurance to cover your worldly possessions!

38% of households with income between $15,000 and $30,000 have a cell phone

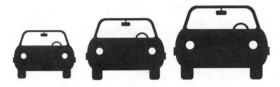

CHEAP   MODERATE   EXPENSIVE

CHAPTER 8
DETERMINING AFFORDABILITY

As you can tell by the number of chapters that deal with cars, there is a lot of information to digest. The fact is that purchasing a car can be intimidating. And the reality is that even though it is the second largest purchase most people make in their lives (buying a house is first), it is typically made *first* in life. But if you take a systematic approach to reviewing the information in the following chapters about how to shop for and buy a car, you should greatly increase your confidence level when dealing with car salesmen and ensure that you don't get "taken for a ride" when trying to purchase a vehicle.

You may know what you want, but the first question most people ask themselves is what can they afford? Apart from your income, there are additional considerations that dealerships and financing companies will use to determine if you can afford your vehicle of choice. How much debt do you have? What is your monthly housing cost? Is your credit top notch, in the toilet, or non-existent? These are all factors that lenders will consider when determining how much financing they will provide.

You can get a general idea of what you can afford based on the information in Box 14.

> The average amount financed in a new car loan is approximately $26,000

Dealerships and salesmen use this formula as an initial guideline to help steer customers to potential cars that are within their budget. Use this figure to calculate your initial budget so you can determine whether you can really afford that new Mustang or if a used Camry is more practical.

BOX 14: CALCULATING AN AFFORDABLE CAR BUDGET		
		Example
Monthly Gross Income		$ 2,000
% for Rent, Car, and Debt	×	40%
Amount Available for Rent, Car, and Debt		$ 800
Less: Rent	–	$ 500
Less: Credit Card Payments	–	$ 100
Monthly Car Budget		$ 200

Before getting to the specifics, as with shopping for a car, you should shop for financing. Talk to a number of banks and ask about pre-qualifying for financing. Based on your income, debt, and other monthly expenditures, many banks and finance companies will be able to provide you with a pre-qualified amount that you can afford to spend. Even if one lender tells you that they are offering you the best rate and lowest down payment possible, check out others. You certainly wouldn't buy a car from the first dealer you visited without checking out others so apply the same rationale to financing. The point is not to limit yourself to the in-house financing arm of the dealer or just the bank where you have your checking account. Shop around.

Car dealerships sold approximately $400 billion worth of new cars in 2002

Let's move on and deal with purchasing a car. If you are going to buy a used car, financing the purchase will prove to be more challenging if you buy one from a private individual rather than from a dealer. The supporting paperwork and validity a bank will need to finance your purchase is more difficult when you buy from an individual. Also, if the used car you are planning to purchase is more than five years old, your financing options will diminish greatly. You should talk to different financing institutions about what supporting paperwork you will need in order to purchase a used vehicle that is not being sold by a dealer.

Typically, you will need to come up with 10% of the final purchase price of the vehicle and will be able to finance the remainder. For example, if the used vehicle you are buying costs $10,000 you will need to be able to pay $1,000 when you close the deal and you will pay the remaining $9,000 over the course of your loan (typically 3–5 years) plus interest charges. For new car purchases, the down payment required can be anywhere from 0%–20% depending upon the vehicle, your financial history, and the lender.

In either case, the term of the loan will greatly impact your interest rate and the total amount you pay over the life of the loan. Don't forget that you are buying an asset that depreciates in value. Simply put, this means that your car is worth less and less as time goes by. Don't get sucked into the lower interest rate on a seven-year loan versus a five-year loan. Beyond having to keep the same car for a longer period of time and incurring additional maintenance costs, you will actually be paying more for the vehicle because of the interest generated on the outstanding balance of your loan.

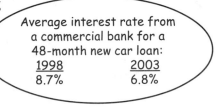

Average interest rate from a commercial bank for a 48-month new car loan:

1998	2003
8.7%	6.8%

There are other factors that impact the deal when evaluating financing options. Understand how much you will need for a down payment, the annual interest rate, the length of the loan, and any additional fees that may apply. The lender should clearly state the total amount of the check you will need to write at closing under a certain deal. Have the lender run various down payment scenarios (e.g., 5% vs. 10% vs. 20%). This will help you in clearly defining your budget based not only on what you can afford on a monthly basis, but also how much cash you can shell out at the time of purchase.

If you are now confused about how much you can afford, don't worry. To assist in determining the monthly cost of various cars under different interest rates, take a look at Box 15 to calculate your monthly payment on a per-thousand-dollar basis.

Box 15: Monthly Loan Cost Per Thousand Dollars Borrowed

Term of Loan

Annual Interest Rate	2 Years	3 Years	4 Years	5 Years
0.0%	$ 41.67	$ 27.78	$ 20.83	$ 16.67
1.0%	$ 42.10	$ 28.21	$ 21.26	$ 17.09
2.0%	$ 42.54	$ 28.64	$ 21.70	$ 17.53
3.0%	$ 42.98	$ 29.08	$ 22.13	$ 17.97
4.0%	$ 43.43	$ 29.52	$ 22.58	$ 18.42
5.0%	$ 43.87	$ 29.97	$ 23.03	$ 18.87
6.0%	$ 44.32	$ 30.42	$ 23.49	$ 19.33
7.0%	$ 44.77	$ 30.88	$ 23.95	$ 19.80
8.0%	$ 45.23	$ 31.34	$ 24.41	$ 20.28
9.0%	$ 45.68	$ 31.80	$ 24.89	$ 20.76
10.0%	$ 46.15	$ 32.27	$ 25.36	$ 21.25

For example, assume you are planning on purchasing a $20,000 vehicle with a 10% down payment (i.e., $2,000) at an interest rate of 7% per year for four years. Multiply 18 (i.e., the amount in thousands that you will be financing: $20,000 − $2,000 = $18,000 ÷ 1,000 = 18) times the number located in the chart corresponding to your term and interest rate.

> The average new car loan from an auto finance company is at 3.6% interest for a period of 63 months

Under this scenario, your monthly payment will be approximately $431 per month (18 × $23.95). If the interest rate is 8%, then your monthly payment will increase to approximately $439 per month (18 × $24.41). Use this chart to calculate how much you can really afford on a monthly basis.

CHAPTER 9
SHOPPING FOR A CAR

B efore getting started, let's back up. Why? Well, most people forget to consider one simple item before going out to the dealerships and shopping for a car. What is it? First, you need to consider *why* you need a car. What will you use it for? Commuting to work? Long road trips? Just cruising the neighborhood? If you carpool or use public transportation, your vehicle needs are vastly different than if you use your car as a part of your job or if you have a forty-mile commute to work each day. Are you really getting a great deal buying an old, cheap ride with 75,000 miles on it if you drive 350 miles each week? There may just be an increased chance it might break down or need major repairs. It doesn't seem like such a bargain now, does it?

Make a list of where, when, and how much you plan to drive your car to begin the selection process. The list will help identify the type of vehicle that will best suit your needs. Regardless of how much car you can afford, clarifying how you will use your car will help you determine if an SUV or compact car is the better option.

Now that you have a clearer idea of the use of your car, let's take a look at the different types and classifications of vehicles.

There are more than 235 million motor vehicles in the U.S.

BOX 16: CAR CLASSIFICATIONS AND COMMON MODELS

Sedans
Chevrolet Lumina
Ford Taurus
Nissan Altima
Toyota Camry
Volkswagen Jetta

Coupes
Chevrolet Cavalier
Chevrolet Monte Carlo
Honda Accord
Honda Civic
Toyota Solara

Convertibles
Chrysler Sebring
Ford Mustang
Ford Thunderbird
Nissan 350Z
Volkswagen New Beetle

Hatchbacks
Ford Focus
Hyundai Accent
MINI Cooper
Volkswagen Golf
Volkswagen GTI

Pickups
Chevrolet Silverado
Dodge Ram
Ford F150
Ford Ranger
Toyota Tundra

SUVs
Jeep Cherokee
Chevrolet Trail Blazer
Ford Explorer
Honda Pilot
Toyota 4Runner

The information in Box 16 provides some different types of cars and their classifications. Even though you likely knew most of this information, it can prove to be a useful list when examining different magazine reports or consumer buying guides for professional evaluations, rankings, and comparisons of different vehicles.

Regardless of whether you are interested in a new or used vehicle, your search will likely lead to at least a few major dealerships. If you have determined that you will be looking exclusively for a used vehicle, there are numerous sources for you to scour in order to find the best car for the best price in addition to traditional dealerships (see Chapter 11: Buying a Car).

In any event, an often-asked question is when to look to get the best deal. Although most salesmen would say that when you shop doesn't make much difference, the fact is that timing could matter when looking for a car. Shop at dealerships towards the end of the month or the end of the year. Why? Well, dealerships are businesses like any other and they all have to try to make their profit numbers on a monthly and yearly basis. Perhaps you will get lucky and hit a dealership that has had a particularly bad month or year. This is just the time when they may be more willing to give you a better deal just to move some cars off the lot. Another good time to shop is in the fall. Dealerships typically start getting next year's model around this time and you can often get some great deals on the current year's model.

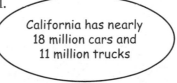
California has nearly 18 million cars and 11 million trucks

Finally, most people work during the week and have to do their car shopping on the weekends. Car dealerships know this so try to search during the weekdays. The fact is that since business is heaviest on the weekends, the best salesmen typically work weekends. And getting the best salesman at the dealership may not always be in *your* best interest. Although shopping at these times certainly does not guarantee a bargain, it could help. It makes sense to try to put any factor in your favor when making such a big purchase.

When it comes to actually visiting the dealerships, use a two-pronged approach. Take one day and visit a number of dealers, ask questions, and test-drive several cars. Even if you are looking for one particular make and model of car, this will give you a sense of the dealership and salesperson you may end up dealing with when purchasing your vehicle. Don't let the pressure of the salesman get to you. His rule of thumb is to not let the potential customer off the lot.

Alaska has only 240 thousand cars and 340 thousand trucks

Again, don't let the pressure get to you. Explain your purpose of the first visit up front; let them know you are shopping around and will not be buying today. They may not like it, but their attitude will tell you a whole lot about how negotiating the purchase will be down the road. If the salesman is aloof and dismissive when you tell him you just want a test-drive and some questions answered, how receptive do you think he will be to knocking a few hundred dollars off the price when you buy the car?

After you visit each dealership, take some notes on the cars you drove using the checklist in Box 17 to narrow your options. Rank each vehicle's attributes, the salesman, and the dealership on a 1–10 scale. Tally up the totals and see where you are likely to get the best deal, best service, and overall positive car-buying experience.

Box 17: Initial Car Selection Checklist	
	Example
Make/Model	Volkswagen Jetta
Car Classification	Sedan
Price	$18,910
Fuel Economy (City/Highway)	24/31
Performance (1-10 scale)	7
Image (1-10 scale)	7
Personal Preference (1-10 scale)	9
Dealership/Salesman (1-10 scale)	6
Notes:	

Now that you have all this in order, it is time to buy a car. You know what kind is best suited for your needs, where to shop for it, and how much you can afford. But there are a number of things you need to understand and prepare before actually purchasing it. Should you buy or lease? What do all the leasing terms mean? What should you look for in a new car? What should you examine when buying a used car? What about insurance rates? These are the types of issues addressed in the following chapters.

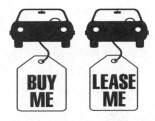

CHAPTER 10
COMPARING LEASING
VS. BUYING

You've decided to get a new car. But should you buy or lease? Which is better? The quick answer is both. Buying a new car or leasing a new car could be the right decision depending on your finances and what you are looking for in a new car.

Let's start with the basics. Unless you have a big pile of cash lying around, both buying and leasing will involve financing. The difference is that if you buy the car, at the end of the financing period you will own the car and can keep driving it until you are tired of it or it gets tired of you and dies. Under a lease, after your leasing period is up, you turn the car back in, have no ride, and must start this whole car shopping experience all over!

However, that doesn't mean that you should automatically buy the car. There are many considerations you should address. How long do you want to drive the same car? Do you like driving a new car every few years? How hard are you on your vehicles? How many miles do you drive in a year? Do you want to drive the nicest car for your money or is that not important? These are just some of the questions you should ask yourself to help you decide whether to buy or lease.

> About 8% of Americans commute one hour or more each way to work

If you drive 25,000 miles a year, beat the crap out of your vehicle, and plan on keeping it for more than five years, then buying the car may be best for you. If you want a new car every few years and want to get the most luxurious car for your money, then leasing may make more sense. The point is that there is no one right answer for every driver. Some people like owning their cars while others don't really care. But you should consider these qualitative factors when making your choice.

Only about 12% of Americans carpool to work

Perhaps the most challenging part of deciding, and often the most important, is the financial difference between buying and leasing. Before examining the differences, consider a few similarities. Whether you buy or lease you will have license fees, sales tax, and other charges due at closing in addition to any down payment you will need to make. Understand all of these costs in each scenario to be sure that you are comparing the numbers correctly.

To directly compare leasing versus buying, Box 18 provides an example under each case to demonstrate the costs involved. Refer to Chapter 12: Leasing a Car for complete definitions of lease terms. Basically, the difference involves the amount of down payment, monthly payments, equity value, and total cost of buying or leasing a car. Often, there will be a larger down payment required to purchase a car than if you lease it.

In the example, you will need to have $2,000 available for a down payment if you choose to buy the vehicle. The lease requires nothing down. This is not always the case, but the lease down payment is typically less than if you buy the car since financing companies will want between 0%–20% down for a purchase. The monthly payments are computed using the same interest rate and term under both scenarios. The payment under the purchase option is higher ($581 per month vs. $344 per month) because you are paying off

The average American passenger car gets 22.1 miles per gallon

both the principle balance of the loan and the interest expenses.

Under a leasing scenario, you are simply paying the amount of depreciation that the car will experience (i.e., the loss in value of the car) during the lease term plus the interest expenses. Once the term of the loan or lease has expired, the equity value represents how much the car is worth to you the buyer or lessee. If you purchased the car, you now own a car free and clear worth $12,500. If you leased it, you own nothing and must turn it back in. Note that the equity value of the car under the purchase scenario is the same amount as the residual value of the car under the leasing scenario. This is simply how much the car is estimated to be worth after three years. Under the leasing scenario, this figure is used to determine the depreciation amount upon which leasing companies charge interest.

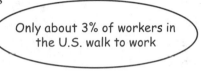

Only about 3% of workers in the U.S. walk to work

Finally, if you look at the total payment less the equity line item, you can see that by purchasing the vehicle, it actually "cost" you less than if you leased it. However, this is simply due to the fact that you are now in possession of a car worth $12,500 versus $0 if you leased the car and have turned it back in.

Just because the total "cost" of buying a car is cheaper than leasing it doesn't necessarily mean buying is better. Do not forget a few key points. First, you forked over $2,000 as a down payment when you would have had to pay nothing down under the lease. Also, you had to pay $581 per month during the last three years when leasing the same car would have cost you only $344. Additionally, you have a three-year-old car that you now must drive and maintain. Finally, if you do choose and sell the car at the end of three years, there is no guarantee that you will get the $12,500 listed as the equity value of the car. For example, if you were only able to sell the car for $10,500, then the total "cost" of buying the car is about equal to the total "cost" of leasing it.

BOX 18: LEASE VS. BUY CALCULATION

LEASING A CAR

	Calculation		Example
	Gross Cost		$ 20,000
−	Capitalized Cost Reduction	−	$ 0
	Adjusted Capitalized Cost		$ 20,000
−	Residual Value	−	$ 12,500
	Depreciation Value		$ 7,500
÷	Term of Lease	÷	36
	Depreciation Component		$ 208
	Adjusted Capitalized Cost		$ 20,000
+	Residual Value	+	$ 12,500
	Total Finance Value		$ 32,500
×	Money Factor	×	0.004167
	Finance Component		$ 136
	Depreciation Component		$ 208
+	Finance Component	+	$ 136
	Monthly Lease Payment		$ 344
	Capitalized Cost Reduction		$ 0
+	Total Monthly Payments	+	$ 12,384
	Total of All Payments		$ 12,384
−	Ending Equity Value	−	$ 0
	Total "Cost"		$ 12,384

BOX 18: LEASE VS. BUY CALCULATION

BUYING A CAR

	Calculation		Example
	Gross Cost		$ 20,000
–	Down Payment	–	$ 2,000
	Adjusted Cost		$ 18,000
	Term of Loan		36
	Amount Financed		$ 18,000
	Interest Rate		10%
	Cost Per Thousand Dollars*		$ 32.27
	*(use chart in Box 15)		
×	# of Thousands Financed	×	18
	Monthly Car Payment		$ 581
	Down Payment		$ 2,000
+	Total Monthly Payments	+	$ 20,916
	Total of All Payments		$ 22,916
–	Ending Equity Value	–	$ 12,500
	Total "Cost"		$ 10,416

The point is that there is no right answer as to whether to buy or lease. It depends on the qualitative factors and desires of the person as much as the finances. However, although the example used compares a purchase with the same terms (purchase price, down payment, term, and interest rate) this is often not the case when shopping for a car. Use the template similar to Box 18 included

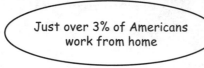

Just over 3% of Americans work from home

in *Real Life 101: The Workbook* to compare the different quotes you get when shopping for a new car. This will enable you to have the financial comparison available in addition to your qualitative needs (e.g., the desire to drive a new car every few years) in order to make the right decision. No matter what people tell you, there is no one best choice. Be clear in you own mind about what you want out of a new car, how long you want to have it, and lay out the financial comparison of buying versus leasing and you will make the best choice for your needs, desires, and budget.

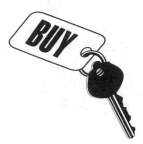

CHAPTER 11
BUYING A CAR

You've determined that buying a car makes more sense than leasing one. Even if you haven't figured out whether to get a new or used car, there are a number of things that you should do to make sure that you choose the best car for you and your transportation needs.

Let's start with buying a new car. Back when you started the whole car shopping procedure, you should have outlined your needs and then narrowed the choices to a few select models or categories of vehicles. Based on your income and other factors you should now know how much you can afford. Yet that still leaves a whole host of cars from which to choose. What to do? As with everything, make a list. Another list?! Yes, this is the only organized way to properly compare key components from vehicle to vehicle to allow you to make an informed decision regarding your new car purchase.

Start with all the features you want and/or need from your car. Do you want an automatic or manual transmission? How important are the safety features of the car? Do you want power locks, seats, and windows? Do you need a two-door or a four-door? What about engine size? Any concerns about fuel efficiency? These are just some of the components that you need to consider

A Porsche 911 GT2 costs $191,700

when deciding on a particular vehicle.

Box 19 provides an example of features that you can use to compare different vehicles during your visits to the various dealerships. Highlight the features that are important to you but make sure to assess all of the areas. You may be surprised to learn that even though you were dead set on having power windows that another model without them surpasses what you thought was your first choice.

Box 19: New Car Features

	Example
Fuel Efficiency	Average
Transmission (Auto or Manual)	Auto
Air Conditioning	Yes
Windows (Power or Manual)	Power
Seats (Power or Manual)	Manual
Locks (Power or Manual)	Power
Mirrors (Power or Manual)	Manual
Cruise Control	Yes
Stereo System	CD
Tires (All Weather Radial)	Okay
Seating Capacity	4
Sunroof/Moonroof	None
Upholstery (Leather or Fabric)	Fabric
Steering Wheel (Adjustable)	Yes
Rust Proofing	No
Trim Package	Standard
Air Bags (Front, Dual, Side)	Front
Traction Control	Yes
Anti-Lock Brakes	Yes

During the test-drive, use the checklist in Box 20 to evaluate how the car felt and handled. Jot down a few notes. You want to be able to accurately compare vehicles when you get home and not rely solely on your memory. Consider all of these factors when making your choice so that you will be happy with the car for many years to come.

Don't forget to write down some information on the costs of each vehicle. Although you likely won't be able to get a final quote from the dealer during your test-drive visit, you should be able to get some idea regarding how much the price will be. This should include what the in-house financing arm can offer you in terms of a loan (e.g., down payment required, fees due at closing, and interest rates). Evaluate this financial comparison

Nearly 17 million new cars, trucks, and SUVs were sold in the U.S. in 2002 along with the features and components of the vehicle to select the best car for your money.

When it comes to actually negotiating the purchase of the vehicle, don't be shy. You know that this is the car for you, but don't necessarily let the salesman know. Be prepared to walk. You've

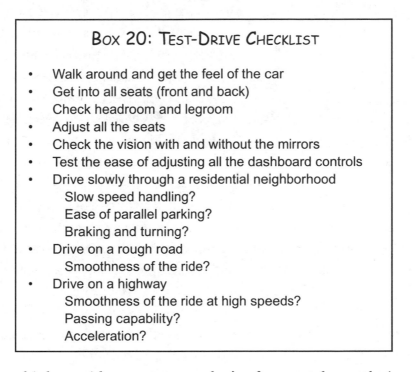

BOX 20: TEST-DRIVE CHECKLIST

- Walk around and get the feel of the car
- Get into all seats (front and back)
- Check headroom and legroom
- Adjust all the seats
- Check the vision with and without the mirrors
- Test the ease of adjusting all the dashboard controls
- Drive slowly through a residential neighborhood
    Slow speed handling?
    Ease of parallel parking?
    Braking and turning?
- Drive on a rough road
    Smoothness of the ride?
- Drive on a highway
    Smoothness of the ride at high speeds?
    Passing capability?
    Acceleration?

gone this long without a new car, what's a few extra days and trip to another dealer to get the best deal on your car of choice! Remember, buying a new car is the second-biggest purchase most people make in their lives (buying a house is the first). Negotiate. You don't have to be an expert negotiator in order to get a good deal, just follow a few key tips.

First, put the odds in your favor and shop at the most opportune times (see Chapter 9: Shopping for a Car). Start by offering to pay 15% below the MSRP (Manufacturer's Suggested Retail Price). You may not get that deal, but perhaps the dealer will agree to 10% or 5% below MSRP. Regardless, try to negotiate at least some discount.

Remember that the dealership makes money on the sale price of the car and on the in-house financing. Even though the salesman will inform you that the dealership and the financing arm are separate entities, the money all flows down to the same company's bottom line. Push the salesman on getting the lowest price, lowest down payment, and lowest interest rate. You also don't want any surprises so make sure he outlines each and every additional charge. What's the worst that will happen? He won't like you. Who cares! You are not trying to become friends with the salesman. Hold firm to what you want in the vehicle and in the price.

There are more than 21,000 new car dealerships in the U.S.

Something else to keep in mind. Dealers are in the business of selling cars. They want to sell you one. Let them. Don't reveal exactly how much you are willing to pay for the car or how much you want to spend on a monthly basis. Be vague; give a range not an exact number. Make them sell you! If you are clear in what you want, how much you want to pay, and take an organized, systematic approach, you'll be able get a good deal on the new car that is perfect for you.

To calculate the monthly cost of buying a car (new or used) use the formula outlined in Box 21. Start with the gross cost of the car (i.e., the negotiated final purchase price). From this, subtract any down payment that you will be making. This is the amount that you will be financing. Refer to the chart in Box 15 to determine which cost per thousand dollars borrowed factor to utilize. In this example, you have a 36-month (i.e., 3 year) loan at 10%. Thus, your cost per thousand dollars borrowed is $32.27.

Texas has 3,234 interstate highway miles, more than any other state

Multiply this amount by the number of thousand dollars you will be financing ($20,000 - $2,000 = $18,000 ÷ 1,000 = 18) to calculate your monthly cost. This particular vehicle under this financing scenario will cost approximately $581 per month ($32.27 × 18). You

Box 21: PURCHASE PAYMENT CALCULATION

	Calculation		Example
	Gross Cost		$ 20,000
–	Down Payment	–	$ 2,000
	Adjusted Cost		$ 18,000
	Term of Loan		36
	Amount Financed		$ 18,000
	Interest Rate		10%
	Cost Per Thousand Dollars*		$ 32.27
	*(use chart in Box 15)		
×	# of Thousands Financed	×	18
	Monthly Car Payment		$ 581

can use this example and the template included in *Real Life 101: The Workbook* to calculate the cost of purchasing various vehicles as you evaluate different options.

Let's move on and address some qualitative factors when considering purchasing a used vehicle. First, there is nothing magical about buying a used car. And there are no guarantees that the car will run perfectly from when you purchase it until you get rid of it. However, there are some guidelines and procedures that you should undertake to help you buy the best used car you can afford.

As with everything in life, if the deal is too good to be true, it usually is. If someone is willing to sell you a car for $500 when the car would typically cost $5,000, who do you think is getting the better deal? If your answer is "the buyer" please contact the

Delaware has 41 interstate highway miles, fewer than any other state

authors of this book since they may have some beachfront property in Nebraska to sell you! There is likely something seriously wrong with the car or it needs constant maintenance. The original $500 could quickly spiral into thousands of dollars just to keep the thing running. The point is simply to be realistic about what you can get for your money when shopping for a used vehicle.

Where can you find a quality used car? There are many places to look. Start with the dealerships. Regardless of whether you purchase a vehicle from one, it will give you a good idea as to the prices of particular models. Look in the newspaper under the classified ads. Check out trade publications focused on selling vehicles. Surf the web. Tell friends and family. You might find out that your friend's friend's grandmother is looking to sell her 1998 Saturn with only 7,500 miles on it for a good price. You never know where you might be able to find the right car at the right price so look everywhere.

What about quality? This is the hard part. Although many cars look good on the outside, they can vary greatly. Some quality used vehicles can be found at dealerships that are called "certified pre-owned." These cars may have a clear record of the owner and maintenance performed.

However, no matter where you choose to purchase the vehicle, there is no better way to assess its quality than to have a checklist of things to look for. Even if you are not a mechanic and don't know anything about cars, there are a number of things that you should examine outside, inside, and under the hood of

New car dealerships sold approximately 19 million used vehicles in 2002

the car. Run your hands over the body of the car and look at the underside of the wheel wells. Are there rough patches in the surface or remnants of different color paint? The presence of either could

BOX 22: USED CAR INSPECTION CHECKLIST

	Examined	Condition
Exterior		
Overall Appearance	√	Good
Body	√	Good
Trim	√	Okay
Paint Job	√	Fair
Rust	√	None
Salt Corrosion	√	None
Windshield	√	Okay
Doors, Trunk, and Hood	√	Okay
Tires	√	Okay
Lights, Brights, Brake Lights	√	Okay
Turn Signals, Wipers	√	Okay
Interior		
General Condition	√	Good
Upholstery	√	Fair
Seat Belts	√	Good
Seats	√	Okay
Windows	√	Okay
Locks	√	Okay
Horn	√	Okay
Dashboard Controls	√	Good
Clock	√	Good
Sound System	√	Fair
Heater/Air Conditioning	√	Good
Under The Hood		
Belts and Hoses	√	Good
Fluids	√	Okay
Oil	√	Low
Battery	√	Okay
Spark Plugs	√	Okay
Air Filter	√	Okay

suggest bodywork or repainting after an accident. Inspect the tires for wear. Check the brake lights, headlights, and turn signals. The last thing you want is to purchase a vehicle only to have to spend additional money to replace worn parts. Look for leaks or puddles on the pavement underneath the car. Check under the hood. This may be as clear as looking at a TV picture

The average price for a used car sold at a dealership was just under $14,000 in 2002

full of snow, but you can identify worn rubber belts and hoses. Ask for the maintenance records of the car. In order to help you check off the items you should examine for yourself, Box 22 provides an example of the exterior, interior, and engine components to review. Test-drive the car on more than one occasion. Note how the car accelerates, turns, handles, and brakes.

Finally, and perhaps most importantly, have a mechanic check the car before you hand over your hard-earned money. You may not be able to do this until close to the end of the deal, but you don't simply want to take the word of the seller that "everything is tip-top." Get an expert's opinion.

Buying a car is likely the largest purchase in your life to date so use your head. Evaluate the car on the facts and not on your emotions. If things don't seem right about the car or the seller, walk away. There are plenty of cars out there in your price range so by using the proper diligence when evaluating potential cars, you'll make an informed, intelligent decision and likely get a great car for a great price.

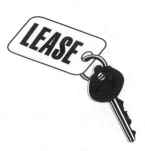

CHAPTER 12
LEASING A CAR

Thinking about leasing a car instead of buying one but unsure what leasing entails? How can you possibly understand all the terms and figures listed on the lengthy agreement? The reality is that this chapter may be the most intimidating chapter in the entire book given the sheer amount of information covered. Car dealerships also seem to keep the particulars of how lease payments are calculated shrouded in mystery. But don't worry, if you take your time and review the information included in this chapter, you will be well prepared when negotiating your new car lease. Believe it or not, it is actually fairly simple and easy to understand once you break down the components of the lease.

Let's take a look at the most pertinent part—cost. There are many terms used when computing the cost of a lease that are unfamiliar to most people. Box 23 provides a list of key terms and definitions that are used in a typical leasing agreement. Using these terms, here is how the cost is determined. First, the overall value of the car (Gross Capitalized Cost) is listed. From this, any down payment (Capitalized Cost Reduction) as well as the value of the car at the end of the lease term (Residual Value) are both subtracted. This result is the amount that you are being

Nearly 2 million vehicles are leased each year in the U.S.

BOX 23: LEASING TERMS

Acquisition Fee – Up-front fee that covers a variety of administrative costs, such as obtaining a credit report and verifying insurance coverage.

Capitalized Cost Reduction – The sum of any down payment, net trade-in allowance, and rebate used to reduce the gross capitalized cost.

Depreciation – A vehicle's decline in value over the term of the lease. This is based on year, make, model, mileage, and overall wear.

Disposition Fee – A "restocking fee" the dealership charges to clean, detail, tune up, and return your car to inventory to sell as a used car when your lease is up.

Excess Mileage Charge – Fee for miles driven over the maximum annual limit specified in the lease agreement. The excess mileage charge is usually between $0.10 and $0.25 per mile.

Excess Wear and Tear Charge – Charge to cover wear and tear on a leased vehicle beyond what is considered "normal." The charge may cover both interior and exterior damage, such as upholstery stains, body dents and scrapes, and tire wear beyond the limits stated in the lease agreement.

Fees and Taxes – The total amount you will pay for taxes, licenses, registration, title, and official (governmental) fees over the term of your lease. Because fees and taxes may change during the term of your lease, they may be stated as estimates.

Gross Capitalized Cost – The agreed-upon price of the car before any down payment, rebate or discount. Think of it as the negotiated "sticker price" for the car.

Lease Term – The period of time for which a lease agreement is written, usually expressed in months.

Money Factor – The money factor is roughly equivalent to the annual interest rate divided by 24. For example, a money factor of 0.00333 equals an annual interest rate of approximately eight percent (0.08 ÷ 24 = 0.00333). Sometimes dealers don't mention the decimal places in a money factor, assuming that you will know that the decimal places are implied. For example, if the money factor is .00333, the dealer might simply say the money factor is "333."

Rent Charge – The financing component of the lease. It is the interest you are being charged to "rent" the car over the course of the lease.

Residual Value – The estimated value of the car at the end of the lease term. It is determined up front in part by using residual value guidebooks but is also negotiable.

charged to lease the car and is often called the Depreciation Value. It's simply a fancy word for the decline in value of the car from the time you drive it off the lot until you turn it back in.

If you simply divide the Depreciation Value by the number of months in your lease, you have the Depreciation Component of the lease. This would be your monthly payment if the dealer decided not to charge you any interest at all. Fat chance!

Only about 1 in 5 car leases is financed by a commercial bank

Here's where wide variations in car leases can occur—the Rent Charge. This is the financing and interest component of a lease and it's where car companies make their money. Rent Charge is the interest you are being charged on the car to "rent" it over the course of the lease.

Take the Capitalized Cost and add the Residual Value of the car to get the total amount on which you will be charged interest (Total Finance Value). Multiply this amount by the Money Factor to determine the total amount of the Financing Component of your lease. The Money Factor is simply the interest rate of the lease divided by 24. For example, an interest rate of ten percent results in a money factor of 0.004167 ($0.10 \div 24 = 0.004167$).

Add the Depreciation Component to the Financing Component and now you have the total monthly lease payment. Box 24 breaks down the lease cost formula to help you in determining how dealerships compute your monthly payment.

Bear in mind that each one of these components is negotiable and will have an impact on the final cost of your car. Be a stickler on all of these points. Try to get the lowest price for the car (Gross Capitalized Cost) and lowest interest rate charged (Money Factor).

The average car lease term is 41 months

If the salesman doesn't have the ability to negotiate the interest charged, then push him on lowering the price of the car. Again, everything is negotiable.

BOX 24: LEASE PAYMENT CALCULATION

	Calculation		Example
	Gross Cost		$ 20,000
−	Capitalized Cost Reduction	−	$ 0
	Adjusted Capitalized Cost		$ 20,000
−	Residual Value	−	$ 12,500
	Depreciation Value		$ 7,500
÷	Term of Lease	÷	36
	Depreciation Component		$ 208
	Adjusted Capitalized Cost		$ 20,000
+	Residual Value	+	$ 12,500
	Total Finance Value		$ 32,500
×	Money Factor	×	0.004167
	Finance Component		$ 136
	Depreciation Component		$ 208
+	Finance Component	+	$ 136
	Monthly Lease Payment		$ 344

Before moving on to the lease agreement itself, there is one more cost item to address—the amount due at signing (see Box 25). Most companies will want your first monthly payment and initial registration fees. There may also be a delivery/acquisition charge along with other up-front fees. Also, this is where the down payment (Capitalized Cost Reduction) will be required. Be sure to cover this information before you get into the room with the finance person to actually sign papers. Don't be excited by a low monthly payment discussed with the salesman only to learn that you have to write them a check for $1,944 upon signing the lease before you can drive off with the car!

Okay, now you know how much you have to pay upon signing the lease and how much your monthly payment is going to be. Let's move on to the other principle components of a typical car lease. First, don't be surprised if the company listed on the top of the lease is a financial institution rather than the car company name (i.e., Chase Bank vs. General Motors). Although many

BOX 25: AMOUNT DUE AT LEASE SIGNING	
	Example
Capitalized Cost Reduction	$ 0
First Monthly Payment	$ 344
Refundable Security Deposit	$ 0
Initial Title Fees	$ 100
Initial Registration Fees	$ 500
Sales/Use Tax	$ 1,000
Acquisition Fee	$ 0
Other	$ 0
Total Due at Lease Signing	$ 1,944

car companies do have in-house financing arms under the same name, some also use banks to provide the financing for their customers. It depends on the dealer and on the qualifications of the buyer as to which financing source is utilized.

Let's address each of the key areas within a lease. The easiest to explain is the length of the lease which is usually expressed in terms of the number of months. For example, a 36-month lease is for three years (36 months ÷ 12 months per year = 3 years). Lease lengths can also be for 48 or 60 months (4 years or 5 years). One "trick" salesmen use is to turn things around and speak of the lease as a three-year lease when in reality it is a 39-month lease and not a 36-month lease. Those three extra months will cost you additional money in terms of total payments and interest rate as well as mean you have the

Financing arms of car dealerships typically finance 4 of 5 car leases

car for a slightly longer time frame. Just be careful when evaluating your lease so that you are clear on the term of the lease. Insist on lease terms in months not years.

Many "great" lease deals are those with much longer lease terms such as 60 months. This may lower your monthly payments, but the interest you pay in the long run will be much greater and you will have to keep the same car for a longer period of time. Decide how long you want the car before being enticed by a lease with a 60-month term instead of one with a 36-month term.

A key factor many people overlook when leasing a car is the mileage they are allowed on a per-year basis. Why is this important? Well, say you go over the mileage limit 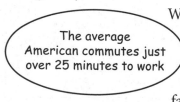 during the term of your lease by 2,500 miles. When you turn your car in, the dealer will politely inform you of this fact and point to the small print in the lease agreement that states that for every mile you exceed the limit, you owe $0.15 per mile. Thus, you will be required to write a check for $375 (2,500 × $0.15) just as you are giving them back your car!

Consider how long your round trip drive to work is everyday and how often you take long road trips. If you aren't sure, find out before you lease a car by tracking the mileage you put on your car for one week (7 days, not just the work week). Multiple this number by 52 weeks and this will give you an idea of your typical annual mileage.

Most leases are given mileage limits of 10,000, 12,000, or 15,000 miles per year above which there is a per-mile fee required at the end of the lease. This fee can range from $0.10 to $0.25 per mile so be sure to add a little cushion to your annual mileage requirement. If you typically drive about 11,000 miles per year, it is better to get a lease allowing 12,000 miles per year rather than try to cut down your driving by 1,000 miles per year. The more mileage you require, the higher the lease cost so balance your driving needs with the associated increased costs.

Now that you know how long and how far you can drive your newly-leased car, you need to address the insurance requirements. To understand the various types of car insurance, take a look at Chapter

The average American commutes just over 25 minutes to work

13: Insuring Your Car. Be clear on the insurance requirements of the lease. Although many states simply require liability insurance to legally operate a motor vehicle, many lease agreements will require additional coverage such as certain monetary levels of bodily injury and/or property damage insurance. Such additional coverage often varies as the type of car you are leasing increases in value (i.e., a Lexus may require more insurance than a Hyundai). You should be clear on what insurance you have currently and if the lease requires additional insurance. The cost of any additional insurance should be taken into consideration when you are calculating how much leasing a particular vehicle will truly cost.

Okay, let's move on to the maintenance of your leased vehicle. Besides simply keeping the car running smoothly, there may be specific maintenance requirements listed in the lease. How often are you required to get an oil change or a complete tune up? Can you take the car to any mechanic or do you have to bring it to the dealer for maintenance? What kind of records will you need to prove that you have kept the car properly tuned? If this information is not specifically mentioned in the lease agreement, ask! Like all other legal agreements mentioned, the car lease may be standard or "boilerplate" according to the salesman, but he does this for a living—you don't. Ask any and all questions you have regarding the lease before signing.

Once the end of the lease term arrives, it's time to turn in the car. If you want to turn your car in before the end of the lease, be advised that there are likely large penalties that you will have to pay. Discuss this possibility with the dealer before signing the lease. But let's go back to the end of the lease term.

3 out of 4 Americans drive alone to work

Typically, there will be a Disposition Fee that you will be required to pay. Think of this as a "restocking fee" the dealership charges to clean, detail, tune up, and return your car to their inventory to sell as a used car. There is not much you can do to avoid this fee but it can often be waived if you chose to lease another car from the dealership.

Also, any excess wear and tear charges will be assessed. These can include any dings and dents or interior damage. It is often advisable when the end of your lease is near to check with your dealer on whether fees will be assessed for certain minor damage and if so, how much. It may make more sense for you to have these imperfections fixed elsewhere before turning in the car since it may be cheaper to do so than to have the dealer charge you. Finally, this is when any excess mileage charges will be assessed.

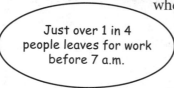

Just over 1 in 4 people leaves for work before 7 a.m.

That is it. You take your car to the location specified by the dealer, review your vehicle for damage, and turn in your keys. Get a copy of the paperwork and confirm with the dealer any charges you will be billed. You don't want to get an unexpected bill six weeks later for a few hundred dollars in excess repair charges.

A final tip when turning in your car: get it washed before taking it to the dealership. Remember how nice and shiny the car looked when you first saw it way back when? You want the inspector to have that same good impression when examining your car for any possible excess wear and tear charges upon turning it in.

If you are planning to lease another car, whether or not it will be from the same dealer, let them know. Car dealerships love repeat customers and will often be very accommodating when assessing any turn-in fees on your old car. Also, they may be willing to give you a "deal" on your next lease since you are a repeat customer. Use the fact that you could be a repeat customer to your advantage when turning in your existing car and when negotiating the lease on your new car. You may just be able to actually get that "great deal" we all hear so much about from car salesman!

CHAPTER 13
INSURING YOUR CAR

You've gotten a great deal on your car and are ready to go cruising down the highway with the top down and the wind blowing through your hair. But just as you are enjoying your first drive in your new ride someone cuts you off and you get into a small fender-bender. No injuries and no major problems—just exchange insurance information and everyone is on their way. Oops! You forgot to get insurance. Okay, so most dealerships and state laws now require that you have insurance before closing the deal, but that doesn't mean that you shouldn't know how to shop for the best insurance and understand what you are getting.

Let's start with an explanation of the different types of insurance (see Box 26). There are a host of supplemental coverage plans that you can have, but most people only need the basics: liability and collision. That said, there are varying degrees of coverage within each category and your state or your financing company, especially when leasing a vehicle, may require certain levels and types of insurance. The dealer should be able to provide you with this information. Ensure that you understand the requirements of your financing company and state.

Liability insurance covers two key areas, bodily injury and property

The economic cost of car crashes was over $230 billion in 2000

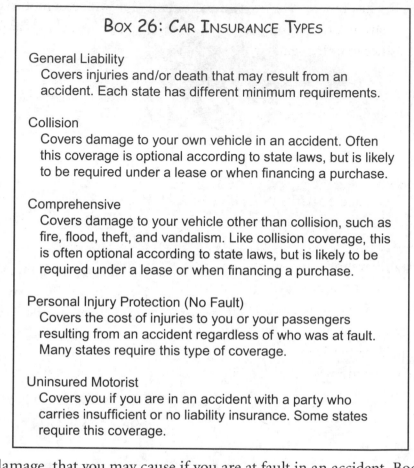

Box 26: Car Insurance Types

General Liability
  Covers injuries and/or death that may result from an accident. Each state has different minimum requirements.

Collision
  Covers damage to your own vehicle in an accident. Often this coverage is optional according to state laws, but is likely to be required under a lease or when financing a purchase.

Comprehensive
  Covers damage to your vehicle other than collision, such as fire, flood, theft, and vandalism. Like collision coverage, this is often optional according to state laws, but is likely to be required under a lease or when financing a purchase.

Personal Injury Protection (No Fault)
  Covers the cost of injuries to you or your passengers resulting from an accident regardless of who was at fault. Many states require this type of coverage.

Uninsured Motorist
  Covers you if you are in an accident with a party who carries insufficient or no liability insurance. Some states require this coverage.

damage, that you may cause if you are at fault in an accident. Body injury insurance covers any medical, pain and suffering, and income loss due to an accident. Property insurance provides a maximum amount paid by the insurance company to the victim of an accident for any vehicle or property damage.

In a typical insurance policy, both types are simply referred to as liability insurance and are often indicated as three numbers such as 25/50/10. This means that the insurance company will pay up to $25,000 per person for any bodily injury you may have caused in an accident, up to $50,000 total for all people involved for bodily injury, plus up to $10,000 to cover any property damage. Many states require liability insurance as the minimum amount of insurance a motorist must have in order to operate a vehicle legally. Confirm your state's insurance requirements with the insurance provider when shopping for car insurance.

Americans drive approximately 2.8 trillion miles annually

Collision insurance has to due with your vehicle and how much the insurance company will pay for damage to your vehicle regardless of who is at fault. Additionally, comprehensive insurance is often listed as part of this type of "physical" insurance that sets a maximum the insurance company will pay to repair or replace your vehicle due to damage from fire, flood, theft, or vandalism. A certain level of collision and comprehensive insurance may not be required by law but is often required when you lease a vehicle.

Other types of car insurance can include uninsured motorist insurance. In an instance when someone without insurance is at fault in an accident, your insurance company pays to have your car repaired rather than trying to collect from the individual who caused the accident. You obtain this coverage because often times it can be difficult, if not impossible, to collect any money from the uninsured individual so it is easier to have your own insurance for this scenario.

Finally, some people choose to add supplemental insurance to cover damages beyond the maximum levels of liability and/or collision insurance. An example is rental car insurance that will provide a rental car, paid for by the insurance company, while your vehicle is out of commission.

The U.S. has nearly 3 million miles of local roadways

All of these types of insurance can prove beneficial in the event of an accident; however, liability and collision insurance are sufficient for most people's needs. Your dealer can provide information about the type and amount of insurance required by law as well as recommended levels. Friends and family are also a good source. Even though everyone you ask may suggest a different amount of coverage, gathering several opinions will aid in your decision for the amount that is right for you.

Once you've determined exactly what types and levels of car insurance you need, the question is where to get it. Chose carefully among the many insurance brokers and providers and don't just pick one at random from the phone book. Hopefully, you will not have to use your insurance company but statistically you will likely be involved in an accident at some point.

This is when insurance coverage matters. The expediency and ease with which you can get a claim paid makes all the difference in the world. The last thing you want to have to do after getting in an accident is to haggle with your insurance company! To this end, it is often wise to choose a company that is 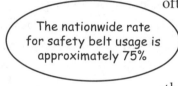 known and reputable. How can you identify such companies? You may already be familiar with several of them. They may be huge conglomerates that provide every type of insurance under the sun including auto insurance. They may also be a specialty auto insurance company with a strong presence in TV advertising. But merely knowing the name doesn't really help.

The only way to evaluate how a company deals with a claim is to talk to someone who's been through the process. Again, family, friends, a coworker, or surely someone you know has been in an accident and could provide you with first-hand knowledge about how the insurance provider handled the situation. The cost for insurance is obviously important but how the insurance company responds is just as relevant.

How much is car insurance going to cost? That depends on a number of factors. It starts with your car. Is it a Volvo wagon or a Corvette? Guess which one is going to cost more to insure? Other factors include your age, sex, and marital status. If you are a young, single male, you pay more for insurance than if you are an older, married woman. This is due to accident rates among males versus females, young versus old, and even single versus married. Additionally, how much you drive your car, where you live, and where you park your car (i.e., in a garage versus on the street) will all factor in determining your insurance rates.

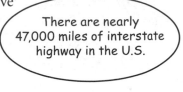

There are nearly 47,000 miles of interstate highway in the U.S.

Since it would be nearly impossible to list all the types of cars and different rates for all the various categories of drivers across the country, the best thing for you to do is to call around for quotes from the group of insurance companies you have selected. Most insurance companies can provide quotes directly over the phone or via the Internet. Don't just go with a company you know nothing about simply because they're the cheapest. Dig around and get a little "inside information" and combine reputation with price to make your selection.

CHAPTER 14
MAINTAINING YOUR CAR

How can you keep your car running smoothly? Simple—maintain it properly. Whether you drive a brand new Honda Accord or a 1984 Chevy Cavalier, the importance of proper car maintenance should not be overlooked. It will help prolong the life of your car, keep the car safe, and even help you get better gas mileage.

Where should you get your car serviced and when? Well, this question is a fearful one for many. Everyone has heard the stories about mechanics overcharging people. How can you avoid this? The only way to find out about a particular mechanic, short of taking your own car in for repairs, is to rely on the experiences of others. You have to ask around and discover the mechanic's reputation. Friends and family members may have an opinion on certain service and repair operations. Seek out a mechanic with a solid reputation. It may cost a little more, but on average, it's money well spent.

The American Automobile Association (AAA) is another great source of information. Consider joining AAA. The group provides emergency roadside assistance anywhere in the country in the event of an accident or break-down. This includes free

> There are approximately 800,000 miles of non-interstate highway in the U.S.

towing to AAA-approved garages. This
can be incredibly helpful should
something happen on a road trip or
outside your local area. The annual
dues are usually around $50 and AAA

New car dealerships performed over 240 million customer repairs in 2002

also provides other services useful to car owners such as maps and
other travel-related information. In any case, AAA can be a valuable
resource when searching for a mechanic. Look for AAA-approved
garages and repair shops.

Aside from an individual mechanic or local garage, consider one
of the national chains. They can provide good service and are often
under more scrutiny by the public and consumer watch groups
simply because they are national chains.

If you are still not sure where to have your car serviced, test
different mechanics and repair shops with simple lube-and-oil jobs.
See how you are treated and how much you are charged. Once you
find a place you trust, stick with it for your routine car maintenance
needs; plus, you'll have the security of knowing where to go should
your car ever need major repairs.

Depending on whether you have a new or used car and where
you bought your car, you may not have a choice in where to go for
service. You may be required to take it to
your dealer or a designated service
provider for regular maintenance
and care. Additionally, many
purchase or leasing agreements have

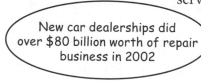

New car dealerships did over $80 billion worth of repair business in 2002

warranties (e.g., 3-year/30,000 miles) that cover routine maintenance
on your car during that term free of charge.

Once you know where to go, the question remains of when to
go and what to have done. Changing your oil every 3,000–5,000
miles may not apply to many of today's newer vehicles as they have
been designed to go longer without an oil change. Also, be aware
that many leased vehicles require various services be performed at

certain time or mileage intervals. Failure to do so can lead to excess wear and tear fees when you turn in your vehicle.

Box 27 provides some of the common car maintenance items and indicates how often you should have these services performed. The different mileage recommendations have to do with how your car is typically driven. If you drive in city stop-and-go traffic or in

Box 27: CAR MAINTENANCE SCHEDULE		
	Frequency	Mileage
Tire Pressure	Monthly	—
Lights	Monthly	—
Lube/Oil Change and Filter	3 Months	3,000 – 7,500
Belts and Hoses	3 Months	3,000 – 7,500
Brakes	6 Months	6,000
Air Filter	6 Months	7,500 – 15,000
Rotate Tires	6 Months	6,000
Wheel Balance	6 Months	6,000
Wheel Alignment	1 Year	12,000

severe hot-and-cold weather, you should have your car serviced more frequently. Ask your trusted mechanic if your maintenance schedule makes sense and refer to your owner's manual. Each car is different and the owner's manual will provide car-specific maintenance information for you to follow.

The bottom line is that regular car maintenance will make both your car and your life run more smoothly.

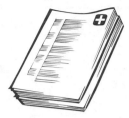

CHAPTER 15
UNDERSTANDING
HEALTH INSURANCE

Y ou are young and healthy so what's the point of covering a topic such as health insurance? Health insurance is something your parents and old people worry about! The truth is health insurance is one of the most important things in your life and is often overlooked or neglected by many young people. Seriously, what is more important than your health? And you better not answer your car!

The fact is getting health insurance and choosing among the various plans can be confusing so it's understandable that many people just take the cheapest option and forget about it. That is until some unfortunate accident or illness occurs and they find themselves at the mercy of whichever healthcare plan they blindly selected. Whether you have to get health insurance on your own (i.e., you're self-employed or your company doesn't offer coverage) or you are covered through your job, you should know the differences in the types of coverage in order to select the best option. To make the topic of health insurance less intimidating, Box 28 outlines some of the basic terms you will encounter when examining your choices.

Each year in the U.S. over $1.2 trillion is spent on personal healthcare expenditures

---

BOX 28: HEALTH INSURANCE BASICS

Premium – The amount you pay for health insurance. It can be paid monthly, quarterly or annually.

Deductible – The minimum amount you pay each year before the insurance company begins paying its portion.

Premium/Deductible Relationship – The lower your deductible, the higher your premiums.

Flexible Spending Account – A special account where you can contribute money before it is taxed. These pretax dollars can then be used for medical expenses such as contacts and prescriptions depending upon your specific healthcare plan.

Co-payment – A small fee you pay for each doctor's visit or prescription under a managed care insurance program.

Primary Care Physician – The doctor you see for regular check-ups and who coordinates and directs all of your medical needs including referrals to specialists.

Network – Under a managed care plan, a group of affiliated doctors and hospitals from which you choose your primary care physician and where you receive your medical care.

Although you may hear various terms used to describe different types of heath insurance, there are basically two types: fee-for-service or managed care. Both cover many aspects of your health including routine medical care, surgical procedures, and hospital expenses. They both may also offer coverage for prescription drugs, dental care, and other healthcare needs. However, there are differences that should be taken into account when selecting the appropriate plan (see Box 29).

First, let's address fee-for-service coverage. This means your doctor or hospital charges you a fee for performing a service such as an annual check-up. Your insurance company covers most of this expense and you pay the other

1 in 6 Americans under age 65 has no health insurance

portion. Often, your insurance company will pay 80% of "reasonable and customary fees for covered expenses" and you are responsible for the remaining 20%. The use of the phrase "reasonable and customary fees" is not an accident. This simply means that if your doctor or hospital charges an amount above what the insurance company has decided is "reasonable and customary" for that particular service, then you will have to come up with the difference.

Box 29: Types Of Health Insurance

Fee-For-Service
Insurance under which you pay a small premium and then only for what services you use. You pay every dollar up to the deductible amount and then your insurance "kicks in." Typically, once you have reached the deductible, the insurance company pays 80% of medical expenses and you pay the remaining 20%.

Managed Care
Insurance under which you pay a higher premium but there is no deductible. Instead, you pay a co-payment amount each time you utilize medical services. The three types of managed care are HMOs, PPOs, and POS plans.

HMO – Health Maintenance Organization. A managed care program that utilizes a network including a primary care physician. To be covered by your HMO, all medical care must be performed by doctors and hospitals affiliated with the network and your primary care physician must refer you to any specialists. When service is provided "in network" you pay only the small co-payment. If you go "out of network" you may be responsible for 100% of the medical expenses.

PPO – Preferred Provider Organization. A managed care program that utilizes a network but does not typically require you to choose a primary care physician. Like an HMO, when you stay "in network" you are only responsible for the co-payment. The difference is if you go "out of network" the program acts like a fee-for-service plan. That is, the insurance company would pay 80% and you are responsible for the remaining 20%.

POS – Point of Service Plan. A managed care program that is a combination of both the HMO and the PPO. Like an HMO, you are required to select a primary care physician. Like a PPO, if you go "out of network" you are responsible for 20% of the costs. Similar to both plans, if you stay "in network" you pay only the co-payment amount.

Your "covered expenses" are those listed in your policy (i.e., the specific procedures mentioned in that big packet of information you got when you signed up for health insurance). Anything other than these covered expenses may fall on you to pay the entire amount. Cosmetic surgery is a typical example of a medical expense that would not be considered a covered expense.

Additionally, under fee-for-service plans, there will be a deductible amount that you will be required to pay each year before your insurance company will begin to pay its 80%. Deductibles can range from $200–$1,000 per year for an individual. Keep in mind that the amount of your deductible will have an opposite relationship to the premiums you pay for health insurance (i.e., the lower your deductible, the higher your premiums and vice versa).

Nearly 30% of adults aged 18-24 have no health insurance

Let's move on to the managed care category of health insurance. There are three major types of managed care service: health maintenance organizations (HMOs), preferred provider organizations (PPOs), and point-of-service (POS) plans.

Under all of these programs, like fee-for-service plans, you pay a premium for coverage on a monthly, quarterly, or annual basis. You will also be charged a "co-payment" for certain services. A co-payment is a small fee associated with each health-related activity. For example, you may be responsible for $15 for every doctor's office visit and $10 for each prescription. There is no deductible to pay and after the co-payment, the insurance company covers the rest.

Under HMO plans, the key component is that you use a doctor or hospital that is part of that particular HMO network. You select a primary care physician that will coordinate all of your medical care and must refer you to any specialists (typically within the HMO network) if needed. Think of your primary care physician as the "quarterback" of your

Over 700,000 doctors currently practice medicine in the U.S.

healthcare coverage. He or she will direct all of your care including referrals to specialist doctors such as a cardiologist or orthopedic surgeon. Thus, choose your primary care physician wisely.

Americans pay for about 17% of health care expenditures out of their own pocket

Typically, a primary care physician is a family practice doctor, internist, or other general care doctor. Some women choose to have their obstetrician/gynecologist act as their primary care physician. The important thing to remember about HMO plans is that if you choose to receive care from a physician or hospital outside the HMO network, then you may be required to cover 100% of the cost of care.

PPO and POS plans operate similarly to HMOs but provide a bit more flexibility. They basically combine the features of HMO plans with that of fee-for-service plans. Both have a network of physicians and doctors that charge you a co-payment for services and insurance covers the rest.

The difference is that if you do choose to receive medical attention from outside the network, then PPO and POS plans operate like fee-for-service plans. Thus, if you go to a doctor outside your PPO network, the insurance company will cover some of the expense (80%) but you will be responsible for the remainder (20%). PPOs differ from POS plans in that under a POS plan, there

24% of adults aged 18-24 visited an emergency room in the past year

is usually a primary care physician (the healthcare quarterback) that will oversee your well-being and refer you to specialists, whereas under a PPO there is not.

Apart from the costs of insurance, the differences in types of coverage will also relate to the medical procedures and care covered. When examining the options, use the checklist in Box 30 to determine what healthcare coverage is provided before basing your decision solely on price.

Also, while some plans will cover dental care, you should be aware that very few plans cover vision care. Instead, some offer a way for you to place some of your paycheck (say $10 per week) before it is taxed into a flexible spending account. That way, rather than using after-tax dollars, you get to use this pretax money to cover items such as contacts and eyeglasses. This is a good idea if you have consistent and predictable expenditures on such items. But be aware that if you don't spend all the money you placed into this account, you will not get it back at the end of the year.

Health insurance is not an easy subject to get a handle on but understanding the basics will help you in selecting the right coverage. Reviewing this information and familiarizing yourself with the different types of healthcare providers will assist you in wading through the documentation associated with any healthcare plan.

The importance of selecting appropriate health insurance based on your needs cannot be overstated so you should ask any and all questions to your benefits coordinator at your job or the insurance company itself before selecting any coverage.

Box 30: Healthcare Checklist

Covered Medical Expenses
- Preventive care and checkups
- Office visits
- Prescription drugs
- Physician visits (in the hospital)
- Inpatient hospital services
- Outpatient surgery
- Medical tests and X-rays
- Physical therapy
- Chiropractic treatment
- Drug and alcohol abuse treatment
- Rehabilitation facility care
- Home health care visits
- Skilled nursing care
- Speech therapy
- Maternity care
- Well-baby care
- Dental care
- Mental healthcare

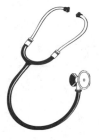

CHAPTER 16
SELECTING A DOCTOR

Regardless of the type of health insurance you select, you will need to choose a doctor, dentist, and eye doctor to keep your health in good order. How do you select a doctor? There are many ways to find qualified professionals such as referrals from co-workers or family and friends, listings in your health insurance information booklet, and even ads in the yellow pages. But apart from whom you select, there is the question of what kind of doctor to select.

To assist you in understanding the different types of medical professionals, Box 31 lists some of the most common types of medical practitioners and a brief description of each. This book cannot tell you which type of doctor is right for you but it provides a better understanding of the types of doctors from which to select when considering all of your choices.

Once you have chosen the proper health care professionals, you should visit your doctor, dentist, and eye doctor on a regular basis. What is a regular basis? Only a doctor can really answer that question so you quickly find yourself in a bit of a "chicken-and-egg scenario." You haven't yet seen a doctor but only your

> The U.S. has nearly 250,000 primary care physicians

BOX 31: TYPES OF DOCTORS

Family Practice – Treats all family members (adult or child) and may include maternity care

General Practice – Provides care not limited to a specialty

Internist – Focuses on nonsurgical diseases in adults

Pediatrician – Oversees care for infants, children, and adolescents

OB/GYN – Specializes in obstetrics and gynecology for women

Opthalmologist – Concentrates on eye disorders and treatment of eye disease

Optometrist – Evaluates visual capacity and fits appropriate lenses

---

doctor can tell you how often you need to see him.

Select a doctor, dentist, and eye doctor, make an appointment to visit each professional for a complete check-up as soon as is practical and then ask the doctor how frequently you should visit him.

If you go for your first visit and don't feel comfortable with that doctor, go to another one. Just because the person is a doctor doesn't mean he or she has to be *your* doctor. Shop around. Many doctors are willing to schedule short, introductory meetings with potential new patients free of charge. While no medical exam takes place, these sessions are a great way to meet a physician and determine if you like a particular doctor. You spent quite a bit of time finding an apartment and shopping for a car, do the same when selecting a doctor. You are now dealing with your most valuable possession— you. Make the choice that is right for you.

Finally, don't take your health for granted and wait until you're ill or injured before seeing a doctor. You're young and in good health. Get in there and see the doctor to make sure you stay that way!

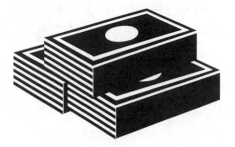

CHAPTER 17
MANAGING YOUR MONEY

S o far most of the topics covered have dealt with various expenses and ways to spend your money. Let's talk a bit about where to keep your money. At this point in life storing your money in a piggy bank, in your sock drawer, or under the mattress is no longer a viable option. You've got to open a bank account if you don't already have one. Specifically, you need a checking account. This is not exactly rocket science, but there is some valuable advice that's worth reviewing.

The reason you need a checking account is pretty straightforward. Instead of carrying around a wad of cash to pay for all your day-to-day purchases, you put your money in a checking account at the bank and then write checks against that account. Pretty simple. At the beginning of the month, you deposit your paycheck and the balance goes way up. Throughout the month, you write checks for all your expenses and the balance goes down. At the end of the month, you're back to where you started so you do the whole thing over again the next month.

87% of U.S. households have a checking account

Okay, most everyone knows this, but what do you really want from your checking account? Obviously, first and foremost is the ability to write checks. When you sign up for a checking account, confirm exactly how many checks you are permitted to write each month. Some accounts have limits as to the number of checks

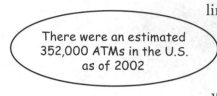

There were an estimated 352,000 ATMs in the U.S. as of 2002

you can write and charge you a fee per check beyond that limit. If this is the case, make sure you're comfortable with the limit or consider an account without a limit.

The next thing you want from your checking account is the ability to withdraw funds from an ATM. Again, this is painfully obvious, but there are still a few types of checking accounts out there that don't have ATM cards linked to the account. Just ensure that your checking account is not one of these old-fashioned accounts. More importantly, inquire about the number and availability of ATMs in your area. You want to make sure there are plenty of your bank's ATMs around. Ask what network your ATM is on (e.g., Cirrus, Interlink, Plus) so when you're traveling or can't find one of your bank's ATMs, you'll know which other banks you can use to access your cash.

Another option to consider when selecting a bank and checking account is the availability of a check card or debit card. Whichever name, the card functions the same way. Basically, the card looks and acts just like a credit card (e.g., Visa or MasterCard), but it actually takes the money directly from your checking account as if you had written a paper check.

Often this check card or debit card is the same card as your ATM card; it just has the Visa or MasterCard logo on it. This feature is free so if you never want to use it, don't worry about, don't use it. But it can come in handy if you're at the grocery store, out of cash, and have forgotten your checkbook. Simply run your card through, type in your PIN, and you're all set. You can even get cash back

A typical U.S. household uses a debit card an average of 7 times per month from the register as if you had made a withdrawal from an ATM. Check cards and debit cards are convenient features of many new checking accounts.

There are approximately 15,000 banks, credit unions, and savings institutions in the U.S.

Another checking account benefit is the advent of electronic banking. The three types are ATMs, banking by phone, and online banking. Although you already use ATMs all the time for withdrawals, you can also use them for deposits, account inquiries, transfers, and basically any other type of transaction for which you would normally visit a human teller. With the exception of withdrawals and deposits, banking by phone allows you to perform all the same transactions as an ATM.

The biggest technological advance is online banking. The benefits of online banking can be great. In addition to being able to monitor your account around the clock and the ability to engage in nearly every conceivable type of banking transaction, you can set up online billing to pay all your monthly bills. There is no need to write a check to the phone company every month when with a few clicks,

The largest bank holding companies in the U.S. are: Citigroup, J.P. Morgan Chase, Bank of America, Wells Fargo, and Wachovia

you can pay the bill online. No checks, no envelopes, no stamps, no hassle! And you'll be able to set up online bill paying for almost every bill you have. You may even be able to set up your account so that your utility company bills are automatically paid each month by having the bill debited from your account when it is due.

There is one other feature you may want to consider when opening your checking account. Many banks offer, and in fact encourage, the use of payroll direct deposit. If your employer is set up for this, you can have your weekly paycheck automatically deposited into your account without receiving a paper check. You no longer need to stand in line at the bank or ATM to deposit it. Plus, if you normally get paid on Friday, often the direct-deposited paycheck hits your account Thursday night at midnight which allows you access to the funds on Friday morning. Additionally, many banks agree to waive monthly fees associated with your checking account if you have your paycheck direct deposited.

Speaking of fees, they often represent a bigger source of differentiation among competing checking accounts than the amenities offered by each account. It's the fees that will usually break the tie when comparing competing banks and account types. Pay attention to the various fees as they can often be the crucial factor in deciding where to open an account.

> There were nearly 14 billion ATM transactions in the U.S. in 2002

The first fee you're likely to encounter is the monthly "maintenance" fee. It may seem absurd, or even offensive, that the bank can charge you a fee to hold your money, but it's actually fairly common. This is particularly true for checking accounts that don't require a minimum balance. The maintenance fee is simply a flat fee per month just to keep the account open. Even if you don't write a single check the entire month, nor do anything with the account for that matter, you still pay the monthly fee. Sometimes this fee can be waived by having your paycheck direct deposited or if you maintain a certain minimum balance.

Maintenance fees are straightforward but there are other fees that are much more difficult to discern at first glance. Some of these fees often seem "hidden" in the sense that they appear to come out of nowhere and pop up unexpectedly on your monthly statement. It's probably unfair to call them hidden, but your bank is not exactly quick to point them out to you especially when you sign up for the account.

> The first U.S. ATM was at Citizens and Southern National Bank in Atlanta, GA in 1971

The best example of this type of fee is the ATM fee, specifically the non-network ATM fee. This is the double whammy that occurs when you withdraw money from an ATM not owned by your bank. Not only does the bank who owns the ATM charge you a dollar or two, but your own bank hits you for an additional one or two dollars as well! This is why it is so important to understand how many ATMs your bank has around town as well as what the bank's fee policy is regarding non-network ATMs.

There are a few other fees you need to ask about when comparing various checking accounts. Certain checking accounts have minimum balance requirements and assess fees should your balance fall below these amounts. Other accounts, particularly those geared towards online banking, impose fees if you transact with a human teller more than two or three times a month. And of course, all checking accounts have the "granddaddy of them all," bounced check fees (in bank language, "Non-sufficient Funds" or NSF). The only way to avoid the monster fees associated with bouncing a check is to avoid bouncing a check altogether.

When opening your new checking account, ask questions as to exactly what benefits and features the account offers as well as

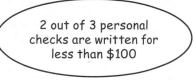

2 out of 3 personal checks are written for less than $100

the minimum balance requirements (see Box 32). Be clear as to what fees are inherent to the account and what fees you could be assessed should you exceed certain parameters. By asking questions and reading the fine print you'll avoid any unnecessary surprises and be assured you're getting the right account for you.

Once your checking account needs are solved, it's worth spending a moment or two discussing savings accounts. In short, there are two versions of savings accounts: a traditional savings account and a money market account.

The traditional savings account is the safest possible place to park your money. You cannot lose money, your funds are insured by the federal government, and you earn interest, albeit at a

```
┌─────────────────────────────────────────────────────┐
│  BOX 32: CHECKING ACCOUNT COMPARISON                  │
│                                                       │
│                                            Example    │
│  Minimum Balance Requirement                $ 100     │
│  Number of Checks Allowed per Month          10       │
│  Check Card/Debit Card                       Yes      │
│  Online Banking Capabilities                 Yes      │
│  Paycheck Direct Deposit Available           Yes      │
│  Monthly Fee                               $ 5.50     │
│  Non-network ATM Fee (per transaction)     $ 1.50     │
│  Human Teller Interactions per Month          2       │
└─────────────────────────────────────────────────────┘
```

remarkably low rate, on your deposited balance.

Money market accounts are not federally guaranteed, could potentially lose value, but offer higher interest rates. Typically there is no minimum balance required for a savings account and no withdrawal penalties. Money market accounts may have minimums and may limit withdrawals.

Neither account is going to make you rich, but if you do find yourself with extra cash, it's worth considering setting money aside for a rainy day in either one of these types of accounts.

A final word when selecting a bank account—the bank itself. You would think that you'd start by picking an institution first and then choose an account type with that bank. Not a bad way to go, but by first determining your needs, it's easier to select the right institution. You have three options.

Average use per ATM was approximately 3,300 transactions per month

First is a small, local bank with perhaps only a few branches in your town. Second is a regional bank with many branches in your town and perhaps throughout your state or neighboring states. Third is a huge, national or international institution with locations throughout a major portion of the United States and perhaps other countries around the world. Which one is right for you depends on what level of service you require.

If you want a basic checking account, prefer to deal with human tellers, and anticipate living in the same area for the foreseeable future, a small, local bank may be right for you. Be aware of the hours of operation of these local banks. One common drawback to these smaller institutions can be limited banking hours during the week or they may not be open on Saturdays. Check with the branch when opening an account.

On the other hand, if you bank online, travel frequently, want a nationwide network of ATMs, and need access to sophisticated financial products, then one of the large, multinational banks could be best. These large institutions may offer extended banking hours and in a few of the largest cities, even have branches open on both Saturdays and Sundays.

As with many decisions, use the information in Box 32 and the template included in *Real Life 101: The Workbook* so that choosing the right account at the right institution will be a snap.

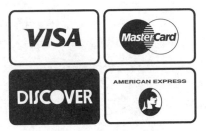

CHAPTER 18
UTILIZING CREDIT CARDS

Well, you've gotten your house in order, found a sweet ride, set yourself up at the bank, and even taken care of health insurance in case you get sick. Life is pretty good. Is there anything you could do to make it even better? Keep playing the lottery, but until you hit the $80 million jackpot you'll likely have to buy a few things on credit instead of paying with that stack of hundreds in your pocket!

Since credit cards have become such a large part of American consumer spending, it make sense to spend a few moments discussing credit cards—the different types, why you want one, and how you get one. Of course everyone knows about credit cards. You may already have one or even two. But it is worth reviewing the topic particularly if you've never been issued a card in your own name.

Although the term "credit card" is thrown around all the time and loosely used to describe any little plastic card that let's you buy things, not all cards are in fact credit cards. The concept of a credit card is simple enough: instead of paying with cash, you pay with your little plastic card all month long and at the end of the month, the credit card company sends you a bill. If you can afford to pay

> Nearly $2 trillion of credit has been extended to individuals in the U.S.

the entire balance in full, great, no interest is charged. But if you can't afford or choose not to pay the entire balance, no problem, the balance carries over and the credit card company charges interest on the amount you still owe. Pretty standard stuff.

The average interest rate on credit card debt is approximately 13%

The key feature of a credit card is the fact that you don't have to pay your bill in full every month. In effect, you're being given a "loan" up to the amount of your credit limit. Basically, if your MasterCard has a $2,000 credit limit, you can spend up to $2,000 of money that you don't have and then pay it off over time when you do have the money.

This is quite different from the other type of card called a charge card. American Express is the most common issuer of this type of card. Although American Express does offer credit cards, the company started off issuing only charge cards, not credit cards. Charge cards look and act almost exactly the same as credit cards with one key difference. You have to pay off your bill in full at the end of every month. There is no option to pay only part of your bill and then pay interest on the outstanding balance. The original American Express "green" charge card (the card featured in numerous print and television advertisements over the years) required every cardholder to pay his balance in full every month and it still operates this way today.

Besides American Express, charge cards are still quite common and are often issued by department stores and specialty retailers.

Credit cards are used more than 12 billion times per year for payments

Sears, Marshal Field's, and Banana Republic are three examples of stores that issue charge cards. The only catch with these type of charge cards is that they are solely for use in their respective stores and can't be used to purchase goods at other stores.

Okay, now you know all about charge cards and credit cards. So why do you actually want one? There are number of reasons to apply for a card and begin using it for at least some of your purchases. The first and most obvious is convenience. Credit cards make purchasing goods and services far easier than using cash or even writing checks. This has always been true for large purchases but with so many merchants accepting credit cards for smaller and smaller amounts, credit cards are replacing checks and cash altogether in many circumstances.

> A typical U.S. household uses a credit card an average of 12 times per month

The Internet is perhaps the best example of why credit cards are convenient, and in fact, necessary for certain purchases. The vast majority of transactions online utilize credit cards. There may be no better reason why you want a credit card than for online purchases.

Another key reason to have a credit card is for travel and reservation purposes. Hotels, car rental companies, airlines, trains, buses, tour operators, and many other travel-related businesses require a credit card for reservations even if you plan on paying by some other method. It's not limited to travel as many gyms, health clubs, and other associations also require credit cards to open an account and to collect monthly dues.

Speaking of travel and reservations, many credit cards have teamed with airlines, hotels, and other businesses to offer a variety of perks just for using the card. These include frequent flier miles, hotel points, purchase discounts on items ranging from automobiles to televisions

> Including credit cards, Americans have over $730 billion of revolving credit available

to groceries, and finally cash rebates. Whatever your interests, there is a credit card available designed to meet your needs.

Even if you're not an online purchaser or don't do much in the way of traveling, having a credit card is still a good idea. A credit card can act as an insurance policy in case of an emergency. If you need to purchase something immediately or find yourself in a short-term cash crunch, a credit card, when used wisely, can be a perfect solution to your problem.

Finally, although not typically considered a benefit by the average credit card user, one of the greatest plusses to having and using a credit card is the positive impact it can have on your overall credit rating. Credit cards as a *positive* impact on your credit? Yes. Of course this implies you have been using the card responsibly and have been paying your bills on time. The fact is, the longer you've had a card and have not been delinquent in your payments, the better your credit record will be. This can be quite valuable when you apply for a car loan or for your first home mortgage.

83% of American households have a credit or charge card

So now you're convinced, you want to have a credit card (or a second or third). How do you get one? Often the best place to start is the very bank where you just opened a checking account. Typically, you'll be able to apply in person when you open the account. If you forgot or that option wasn't available, your bank should have applications available at the branch, by phone, or online.

If your own bank does not approve you, don't despair, there are still other options. The next step is to apply to one of the large, multinational banks such as Chase, Bank of America, or Citibank. Even if one of these larger institutions isn't right for your checking account needs, it may be right for your credit card needs.

Nearly half of U.S. households carry a credit card balance

There are also a number of credit card issuers who, while not traditional banks with individual branches, specialize in issuing credit cards and are among the most aggressive in attracting new card members. Two of the largest are Capital One and MBNA. Both companies have a strong Internet presence and allow you the opportunity to apply online as well as by phone or by mail. Box 33 provides an example of some typical credit card features that should be evaluated.

Box 33: Credit Card Account Comparison

	Example
Annual Fee	$ 50
Introductory Interest Rate	2.99%
Length of Introductory Period	6 months
Long Term Rate (following intro period)	14.99%
Transfer Balances onto New Card	Yes
Balance Transfer Fee	3% of amount transferred
Perks (e.g., mileage program)	American Airlines Miles

Don't forget about the charge card option either. Even if you ultimately desire to have a credit card, getting a charge card first is not a bad way to go. Once you get the charge card, use it for a few months making routine purchases and paying off the balance in full at the end of each month. This cycle of charging followed by timely payment is positively reflected in your credit report and often leads to credit card issuers contacting you directly asking you to apply for one of their cards. Using a charge card in small doses for several months can sometimes be the best way to establish a credit history if you don't already have one.

Remember that a charge card doesn't have to be from American Express or another financial institution. Store-sponsored charge cards are another way to establish a solid credit history. Although these store cards often have low credit limits and are only usable for purchasing goods in their respective stores, they often have much lower qualification requirements than a typical charge or credit card and still provide a great way to establish good credit.

If you've struck out completely so far, there are still other options. One of the most common ways for you to get a credit card in your own name when you cannot qualify is to have someone cosign with you.

This person, the cosigner, uses his credit history to be approved by the bank. Although the card is in your name and not his, the cosigner is still legally responsible for all charges. The cosigner agrees to step in and assume the debt in the event that you fail to make payments. Your parents or other relatives are the most likely cosigners but you do not necessarily have to be related to the person who cosigns on your behalf.

79% of American households receive monthly offers to apply for a credit card

Once you have the card for several months and have established a good payment history, you can contact the credit card company and ask to have the cosigner removed and you can take over sole responsibility for your own credit card.

Another option is to go the route of the secured credit card. Up to this point, every reference to credit cards has been to unsecured credit cards. Typically, when you are approved for a credit card, you provide no collateral (i.e., guarantee of payment) in return for the credit that is extended to you other than your promise to pay. This type of card is therefore unsecured. This works great for those with good credit.

However, if you have no credit history, banks are often reluctant to issue you this type of credit card since they have no guarantee that you will, in fact, pay. This creates another "chicken-and-egg scenario." You have no credit history, so no one wants to issue you a credit card, but without a card, you'll never be able to establish a credit history.

Enter the secured credit card. It's exactly the same as a traditional

45% of U.S. households have a store charge card

credit card except that you "secure" the card by providing collateral to the bank. Specifically, you actually prepay money to the credit card issuer. If you want a Visa card with a $300 limit, you send $300 to the bank and the bank then issues you a "secured" Visa card.

Remember, your goal with this type of card is not to create huge purchasing power, but merely to establish as quickly as possible that you can be responsible with the card and will pay your bills on time. Once you have the card, steer some of your purchases for which you would normally pay cash onto the card (groceries are a great example) and then immediately pay off the charged amount.

Store cards are used more than 2.7 billion times per year for payments

Demonstrating a pattern of charges followed by prompt payment in full is exactly the credit history you want to establish with your card provider. After a few months, contact the issuer and request the return of your secured amount and switch the card from secured to unsecured. Continuation of this same responsible purchase/payment pattern will also allow you to request an increase in your credit limit. As with the charge card, once you've established a solid credit record with the secured card, you'll be surprised how many credit card companies may offer you one of their unsecured cards.

No credit card discussion would be complete without mentioning the potential dangers associated with accessing lines of credit. First and foremost, credit cards are *not* a source of free money! Although they may appear to be, don't be fooled. Whatever your credit limit, you are responsible for each and every dime you put on the card.

Don't go on a wild shopping spree or purchase a series of gifts for yourself without a thought of the consequences. It is very easy for debts to spiral out of control. Once you start falling behind on monthly payments, the high interest rates and compounding factor of the interest can easily cause your debt to increase significantly. You need to scrutinize all of the purchases you make with your credit cards. A credit card is supposed to be a convenience tool to allow you simply to use plastic instead of cash. In other words, it's a good

The average store card charge is $59

idea only to make purchases on the card that you would otherwise make with cash. Too many people still make all their normal purchases with cash or by check and then use their credit card for additional purchases of luxury items. This is a risky proposition that can be detrimental to your current and future financial situation.

Another fact that many people are not aware of is that the amount of credit you are granted by each issuer is counted as part of your total amount of credit regardless of whether you use it. For example, if you have a Visa with a $3,000 credit limit and a MasterCard with a $2,000 limit, your credit report will show the total $5,000 available credit even if your outstanding balance on those cards is only $350. Separate from your outstanding balances, other credit issuers (e.g., car dealership finance arms) will factor this information in when evaluating you for a car loan. Therefore, be careful when and where you decide to gain credit.

Americans use credit cards and charge cards to spend over $1 trillion per year

Also, if you decide that you no longer want a particular credit card or wish to decrease the total amount of credit extended to you, simply cancelling the card is not enough. You need to take the extra step and contact the credit reporting agency directly and have them remove this credit amount from their records as well. Just cancelling your card while in good standing with Visa or MasterCard is not sufficient. When cancelling the card, ask the provider whom to contact to remove the credit amount from your credit record entirely.

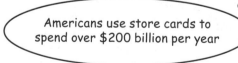

Americans use store cards to spend over $200 billion per year

Furthermore, if you damage your credit record by overspending, making late payments, or by failing to make payments altogether, there can be lasting implications. Once you've established a negative credit history, it can be a very difficult hole from which to dig yourself out. Just as establishing a good credit history can enhance your chances for a car loan or home mortgage, poor credit can hamper your chances to qualify for these major loans later in life.

When used responsibly, credit cards are an excellent financial tool that can make your everyday life easier, more efficient, and more convenient. The important thing to remember is to spend responsibly, keep detailed records of your purchases, and pay your bills on time.

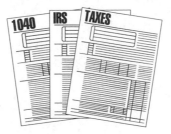

CHAPTER 19
DOING YOUR TAXES

Doing your taxes is probably the least fun topic in this entire book. But as much as you might not want to pay taxes, you still have to. For many people though, what is worse than paying taxes is actually doing their taxes, i.e. filling out all the government paperwork. It may be painful but there are things you can do to make the ordeal manageable.

Most people know that income taxes are due once a year on April 15th. You have to pay taxes both to the federal government and to the state in which you live. You may also have to pay local income taxes as well if you live in a major urban area such as New York City. Whatever the case, this means there are plenty of forms to fill out during the first half of April.

The biggest problem people have when doing their taxes is time—specifically, lack of it. Too many people so dread doing their taxes that they wait until the last possible minute and then rush to get everything done before the filing deadline. Do this and you've just compounded the problem. Take something you already don't want to do and then add time pressure and stress to it—not a good combination.

Even though taxes aren't

> The IRS collected more than $1 trillion in individual income taxes in 2002

due until April 15th, there are plenty of things that can be done long before then to simplify the process.

First, what forms do you actually need in order to do your taxes? What paperwork should you gather? What should your employer give to you? Where should you get everything? The first piece of paper you need to worry about is what is

Over 30,000 people in California earned more than $1 million in 2002

called a "W–2" or a "Form W–2." You can't do your taxes without a W–2 since this form tells you how much tax the government has taken out of your paycheck each week for the previous year. You have to start here in order to figure out if you've paid too much and the government owes you a refund or if you've paid too little and you owe the government.

Remember the form you filled out when you started your job and indicated the number of dependents you claim? This was the basis used to determine how much tax was taken out of your paycheck throughout the year. For a single person, selecting one or more dependents meant that less tax was taken out during the year (thus increasing your weekly paycheck) and you may find yourself owing money to the government at the end of the year. Conversely, if you selected zero dependents, then more taxes were subtracted from your paycheck during the year and you may be entitled to a refund of any excess taxes that you paid. When filling out your paperwork at a new employer, be sure to balance your day-to-day financial needs with your year-end tax responsibilities. Ask someone in your employer's human resources department for details on how your selection will impact your weekly pay and your year-end tax situation.

Only 132 people in North Dakota earned more than $1 million in 2002

Your W–2 will be given to you by your employer. By law, the employer has to issue W–2s to all employees by the end of January.

For example, W–2s for 2004 will be distributed no later than January 31, 2005. So with taxes for 2004 not due 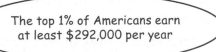 until April 15, 2005, you have at least two and a half months to do your taxes before the deadline. There is absolutely no need to compute your taxes at the last possible minute.

Okay, you have your W–2, now what? Time to get the government forms (see Box 34). For federal filing you'll need either Form 1040 or Form 1040EZ. Form 1040 is the standard form that most people in the country can use to do their taxes. Form 1040EZ is a shortened, single page version that makes it easier (hence the name) and simpler

---

Box 34: Tax Preparation Documents

W-2 – Recap of annual gross income and all taxes paid

1040 – Standard federal income tax form that can be used by most people in the country

1040EZ – Single page, short form that can be used by singles and married couples filing jointly with less than $50,000 income

1099-INT – Statement of interest income from savings or investment accounts

1099-DIV – Statement of income received from dividends or capital gains on shares of stock

1099-G – Statement of unemployment income

1099-MISC – Statement of miscellaneous, other income

---

for the individual. Most people starting out on their own who are single or married filing jointly are eligible to use the EZ form. The exceptions are people who have bought and sold shares of stock or bonds during the year and have capital gains and losses, people who itemize individual tax deductions instead of taking the standard deduction, and those with earnings greater than $50,000.

For the purposes of this book, it's assumed that most readers fall into the EZ category. The forms

> The top 10% of Americans earn at least $92,000 per year

themselves and the instruction booklet outline the qualifications of which form to use so double check to ensure that you are using the proper form. If there is any doubt, use the standard Form 1040. You'll figure your taxes exactly the same regardless of which form you use; it's merely a question of time and convenience.

You'll also need to get the form for your state income taxes. The name or number of this document varies by state so you have to check with your home state to get the proper form. In nearly every state it's a single page since many of the required calculations have already been done on the federal forms.

There are several options as to where to get both the state and federal forms. Beginning in January, the post office and municipal libraries have all necessary federal, state, and local forms available in the lobby or at a designated area. If you filed taxes the previous year, the government usually mails you the proper forms and instruction booklet; but just in case, stop by the post office or library. Federal forms and most state forms are also now available online and can be downloaded and printed at home. Contact the Internal Revenue Service at *www.irs.gov* for the proper forms. Most states have the forms available on the Internet as well so check your state's website.

It's early February, you have your W–2, your federal Form 1040EZ, your state form, and the corresponding instruction booklet. Time to actually do your taxes. Since you're so far in front of the April 15th deadline, use the time to your advantage. Pick a rainy weekend, a quiet evening, or a random Tuesday night and set it aside as the time to do your taxes.

By scheduling time, you won't feel rushed and there's no pressure to get everything done in one sitting. If you've given yourself a migraine headache after two hours of number crunching, call it a day and go back to it later. That's the beauty of starting weeks or months in advance. Plus, the earlier you start, the earlier you finish. If the government owes you a refund, it'd be nice to get that check in early March as opposed to late May. On the flip side, even if you owe the government, you can still wait until April 15th to mail the check. You just won't be scrambling around at the last minute. Your taxes will already be done; you're simply hanging on to your money a little while longer.

If you're using the EZ form, all you really need to do your taxes is your W-2, a pen, and a calculator. That's it. Even though the government writes it, the instruction booklet actually does a good job of walking you through the process line item by line item. You don't have to be a math wizard or an accountant to do your own taxes. Always do your federal income taxes first because in order to fill out the state forms, you'll need to have already completed the federal form.

You may also choose to purchase electronic tax preparation software (e.g., Turbo Tax). These programs are relatively inexpensive and make doing your taxes even easier. Plus, if you utilize electronic organization software such as Quicken or Microsoft Money, the tax program can even pull much of the necessary information directly from these programs which simplifies the process even further.

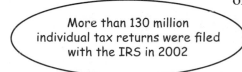

More than 130 million individual tax returns were filed with the IRS in 2002

Life gets more complex if you've got a vast stock portfolio or itemize individual deductions. It's beyond the scope of this book to discuss those scenarios here. Suffice to say is that you'll definitely be filling out Form 1040 and will need several other forms and related paperwork in order to complete your taxes.

Additional papers, documents, and receipts aren't really

necessary in order to do your taxes; they only come into play in the unfortunate event of an audit by the IRS. Being audited is an inconvenience but doesn't necessarily mean you've done anything wrong. The IRS conducts thousands of random audits every year just to ensure people are completing their tax forms properly and everyone is paying their fair share.

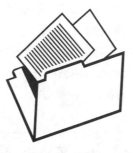

CHAPTER 20
ORGANIZING PAPERWORK

If you haven't already learned that the adult world involves a heck of a lot of paperwork, you soon will. Just think about the paperwork you already have: apartment lease, car purchase or lease agreement, car insurance forms, health insurance information, monthly bank statements, credit card bills, ATM withdrawal slips, credit card purchase receipts, etc., etc., etc. And guess what? It only gets worse as your life gets more and more complicated.

How do you organize all of this information? You could choose the shoebox method but what happens when you need the receipt to return something? What about if you need to check whether you paid a bill or not? Do you really want to spend an afternoon pouring through a box of clutter? Even if you do everything on your computer (such as manage your checking account or pay bills) you would be surprised how quickly things can get disorganized and out of hand. Let's not even address the potential hazards for those of you who just throw everything away.

Believe it or not, it is actually easy to get organized, and more importantly, even easier to stay organized if you set up your record-keeping in a systematic

> The United States Postal Service delivered nearly 203 billion pieces of mail in 2002

fashion. And the best part is once you have this system set up you won't even have to think about it!

Let's start with the one thing that you have to do on a monthly basis—pay bills. You should start by making a list of all of your monthly bills and their respective due dates. Box 35 provides an example of a master schedule. When it is time for you to pay a bill,

Box 35: Monthly Bills Checklist

	Due Date	Example Jan.
Rent	1st	$ 500.00
Car Payment	30th	$ 225.45
Car Insurance	30th	$ 70.75
Health Insurance	30th	$ 121.51
Phone	15th	$ 24.75
Electricity	28th	$ 17.95
Cable	15th	$ 34.50
Internet	15th	$ 20.95
Water	30th	$ 12.95
Gas	30th	$ 14.10
Cell Phone	28th	$ 35.00
Credit Card #1	28th	$ 50.00
Credit Card #2	19th	$ 75.00

simply record the amount paid for that particular month. By using this master schedule you'll never forget to pay the phone bill since it will be listed right there in front of you. Plus, you can avoid late payment penalties by paying the bill on time even if the bill got lost in the mail and you never received it. Bottom line, do you really want to rely on your memory to ensure that you pay all your bills? Write out a schedule ahead of time.

Okay, so you can pay your bills on time, but what about all that paperwork? This is where the "manila folder method" earns its keep.

The best way to stay organized is to create a separate manila folder for each monthly bill and keep all the folders in a file cabinet or closet. You could use regular envelopes, but these tend to get bulky and cumbersome since different bills are different sizes.

Start out by making a folder for each line item on your master schedule (e.g., phone, power, cable, etc.). Then create a

The majority of American households receive an average of 5 credit card offers per month

master "Monthly Bills" folder and put each of the monthly bills in this folder as they come in during the month. Then when it comes to "bill-paying night," empty the master Monthly Bills folder, write a check for each bill, record each payment on the master schedule, and re-file these bills into their respective individual folders. You end up with every bill paid for that month and an empty (until next month) Monthly Bills folder. This isn't exactly rocket science, but how many people do you know have all this information easily accessible and organized? Trust this system. It works.

What about all the credit card and ATM receipts you get every day or week? No real difference from your bills. Simply have a separate folder for each credit card or bank account and put the receipts in those folders as you get them. Obviously, the key to this is actually keeping the receipts. And don't be ridiculous, it really isn't that hard to keep these receipts in your wallet or purse until you get home at night!

At the end of the month, you can easily reconcile (i.e. compare the issuer's records to your own) bank statements and credit card bills to be sure that only your withdrawals and the items you charged are

Americans wrote 42.5 billion checks in 2000

listed. Plus, simply from the number of receipts in your files, you will start to get an idea as to how much money you are going through on a monthly basis. Once you reconcile your monthly bank and credit card statements, just staple the corresponding receipts to the back of each statement and you're done for that month.

It really doesn't take much time and now you have a complete record of all of your withdrawals and charges. Should you have a charge on your credit card that you don't recognize, you will be able to inform the credit card issuer that you keep all the receipts from your charges and you don't have this one. It will greatly enhance your ability to have these charges removed from you bill and ensure that you are not responsible for incorrect charges. And let's not forget how handy these receipts and records will be in the unlikely and unpleasant event of an IRS tax audit!

You've reached the end of the year and you have all these manila folders with bills for each month, receipts stapled to each month's bank and credit card statement, and a completely filled-in master schedule. What now? Start over. Make another blank master schedule and manila folder for each line item.

Gather all the previous year's folders and put them into a box and store in your closet. Why can't you throw them away? First of all, you may need to refer to some of this information when you are filling out your tax forms and also because the IRS does recommend that you keep such records for the last three years. They won't take up that much space. That's it. You have last year's records stored and a bunch of empty folders to begin your second year of organized, hassle-free living!

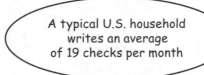

A typical U.S. household writes an average of 19 checks per month

A brief word on electronic organization. There are programs such as Quicken and Microsoft Money that can organize all your banking, credit card, and other accounts and also provide easy reconciliation and monthly reminders. These are great programs and are relatively simple and easy to use. Also, many people receive online bills instead of paper bills or use scanners to store all their financial information on their computer. But even if you do store all your information electronically, you should still apply the manila folder methodology and organize all your electronic bills and information into different file folders. Even though your computer is an excellent way to organize your information, it does not totally negate the use of the physical manila folder method to keep track of all the paperwork you receive. Some companies still send paper bills through the mail even if they have electronic bill payment. Whether or not you use your computer, you will still need to keep your paper files organized.

Credit card issuers send out approximately 5 billion solicitations per year

Now that wasn't so bad, was it? The point is that since you have made such informed, sound decisions regarding your apartment, furnishings, car, health insurance, banking, and credit card usage, it doesn't make sense to keep the records of your good decisions in disarray. Don't add undo hassle to your life. You have plenty to concern yourself with without worrying about where your bank statements are or if you paid your bills on time.

Make your life run more smoothly by keeping yourself organized now when things are relatively simple and easy to track. Life only gets more complicated (and fun) when you start buying a house, getting married, having kids, saving for retirement, and so on. But those are topics addressed in the next book…

...XYZ

CONCLUSION

T he goal of this book has been to present many of life's day-to-day challenges in a less intimidating manner and to assist you in making sound decisions. The examples included in the information boxes were provided to increase your understanding of each topic in order to make the relevant decisions even more straightforward. Even if you didn't utilize all the tips and tactics outlined in each chapter, hopefully you learned something that helped make at least one decision regarding your home, car, healthcare, or finances easier and less stressful.

Don't worry if you didn't follow all the information provided or even if you made some mistakes along the way. At least you improved your *Trivial Pursuit* skills by taking a look at the fun fact ovals spread throughout the book! The knowledge presented in this book was gained through a series of missteps and misjudgments regarding the very topics covered in each chapter. Learn from the authors' mistakes so that you can minimize your own. You won't be able to make perfect choices in every facet of your life, but hopefully the book provided you with the essential information to avoid some common pitfalls.

Use the information in this book in conjunction with *Real Life 101: The Workbook* to create your own decision-making templates as you are confronted with life's everyday choices.

The bottom line is that armed with the material and information included in *Real Life 101*, you now have *A Guide To* assist you and should be confident in your ability to make informed decisions on *Stuff That Actually Matters*.

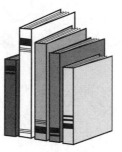

SOURCES

Page 15. U.S. Department of Commerce. U.S. Census Bureau. Census 2000. *Housing Costs of Renters: 2000.* May 2003.

Page 16. U.S. Department of Housing and Urban Development. U.S. Department of Commerce. U.S. Census Bureau. *American Housing Survey for the Phoenix, AZ Metropolitan Area: 2002.* July 2003.

Page 17. American Honda Motor Co., Inc. Official Company Website. *www. honda.com.* December 2003.

Page 17. U.S. Federal Reserve Board of Governors. Federal Reserve Bulletin. *The Use of Checks and Other Noncash Payment Instruments in the United States.* August 2002.

Page 18. U.S. Department of Education. National Center for Education Statistics. *Digest of Education Statistics 2002.* June 2003.

Page 19. U.S. Department of Labor. Bureau of Labor Statistics. *Occupational Outlook Handbook, 2002–2003 Edition.*

Page 21. U.S. Department of Housing and Urban Development. U.S. Department of Commerce. U.S. Census Bureau. *American Housing Survey for the Anaheim–Santa Ana, CA Metropolitan Area: 2002.* July 2003.

Page 23. U.S. Department of Housing and Urban Development. U.S. Department of Commerce. U.S. Census Bureau. *American Housing Survey for the Buffalo, NY Metropolitan Area: 2002.* July 2003.

Page 23. U.S. Department of Housing and Urban Development. U.S. Department of Commerce. U.S. Census Bureau. *American Housing Survey for the Charlotte, NC–SC Metropolitan Area: 2002.* July 2003.

Page 24. U.S. Department of Housing and Urban Development. U.S. Department of Commerce. U.S. Census Bureau. *American Housing Survey for the Columbus, OH Metropolitan Area: 2002*. July 2003.

Page 24. U.S. Department of Housing and Urban Development. U.S. Department of Commerce. U.S. Census Bureau. *American Housing Survey for the Milwaukee, WI Metropolitan Area: 2002*. July 2003.

Page 25. U.S. Department of Housing and Urban Development. U.S. Department of Commerce. U.S. Census Bureau. *American Housing Survey for the Dallas, TX Metropolitan Area: 2002*. July 2003.

Page 26. U.S. Department of Housing and Urban Development. U.S. Department of Commerce. U.S. Census Bureau. *American Housing Survey for the Kansas City, MO–KS Metropolitan Area: 2002*. July 2003.

Page 28. U.S. Department of Housing and Urban Development. U.S. Department of Commerce. U.S. Census Bureau. *American Housing Survey for the Portland, OR–WA Metropolitan Area: 2002*. July 2003.

Page 29. U.S. Department of Commerce. U.S. Census Bureau. March 2000. Current Population Survey. *Geographical Mobility: March 1999 to March 2000*. May 2001.

Page 30. U.S. Department of Commerce. U.S. Census Bureau. March 2000. Current Population Survey. *Geographical Mobility: March 1999 to March 2000*. May 2001.

Page 30. U.S. Department of Commerce. U.S. Census Bureau. March 2000. Current Population Survey. *Why People Move: Exploring the March 2000 Current Population Survey*. May 2001.

Page 32. U.S. Department of Commerce. U.S. Census Bureau. March 2000. Current Population Survey. *Geographical Mobility: March 1999 to March 2000*. May 2001.

Page 32. U.S. Department of Commerce. U.S. Census Bureau. March 2000. Current Population Survey. *Geographical Mobility: March 1999 to March 2000*. May 2001.

Page 33. U.S. Department of Commerce. U.S. Census Bureau. March 2000. Current Population Survey. *Why People Move: Exploring the March 2000 Current Population Survey*. May 2001.

Page 33. U.S. Department of Commerce. U.S. Census Bureau. March 2000. Current Population Survey. *Geographical Mobility: March 1999 to March 2000*. May 2001.

Page 34. U.S. Department of Commerce. U.S. Census Bureau. Census 2000. *Housing Costs of Renters: 2000*. May 2003.

Page 34. U.S. Department of Commerce. U.S. Census Bureau. Census 2000. *Housing Costs of Renters: 2000*. May 2003.

Page 35. U.S. Department of Commerce. U.S. Census Bureau. Census 2000. *Geographical Mobility: 1995 to 2000.* September 2003.

Page 36. Department of Commerce. U.S. Census Bureau. Census 2000. *Geographical Mobility: 1995 to 2000.* September 2003.

Page 37. Department of Commerce. U.S. Census Bureau. Census 2000. *Geographical Mobility: 1995 to 2000.* September 2003.

Page 39. U.S. Department of Commerce. U.S. Census Bureau. March 2000. Current Population Survey. *Why People Move: Exploring the March 2000 Current Population Survey.* May 2001.

Page 40. Department of Commerce. U.S. Census Bureau. Census 2000. *Geographical Mobility: 1995 to 2000.* September 2003.

Page 40. Department of Commerce. U.S. Census Bureau. Census 2000. *Geographical Mobility: 1995 to 2000.* September 2003.

Page 42. Department of Commerce. U.S. Census Bureau. Census 2000. *Geographical Mobility: 1995 to 2000.* September 2003.

Page 42. Department of Commerce. U.S. Census Bureau. Census 2000. *Geographical Mobility: 1995 to 2000.* September 2003.

Page 43. U.S. Department of Energy. Energy Information Administration. 2001 Residential Energy Consumption Survey. *The Effect of Income on Appliances in U.S. Households.* November 26, 2002.

Page 44. U.S. Department of Commerce. Economics and Statistics Administration. National Telecommunications and Information Administration. *A Nation Online: How Americans Are Expanding Their Use of the Internet.* February 2002.

Page 44. U.S. Department of Commerce. Economics and Statistics Administration. National Telecommunications and Information Administration. *A Nation Online: How Americans Are Expanding Their Use of the Internet.* February 2002.

Page 45. U.S. Department of Commerce. Economics and Statistics Administration. National Telecommunications and Information Administration. *A Nation Online: How Americans Are Expanding Their Use of the Internet.* February 2002.

Page 46. U.S. Department of Commerce. Economics and Statistics Administration. National Telecommunications and Information Administration. *A Nation Online: How Americans Are Expanding Their Use of the Internet.* February 2002.

Page 47. U.S. Department of Energy. Energy Information Administration. 2001 Residential Energy Consumption Survey. *The Effect of Income on Appliances in U.S. Households.* November 26, 2002.

Page 48. U.S. Department of Energy. Energy Information Administration. 2001 Residential Energy Consumption Survey. *The Effect of Income on Appliances in U.S. Households.* November 26, 2002.

Page 48. U.S. Department of Energy. Energy Information Administration. 2001 Residential Energy Consumption Survey. *The Effect of Income on Appliances in U.S. Households.* November 26, 2002.

Page 50. U.S. Department of Energy. Energy Information Administration. 2001 Residential Energy Consumption Survey. *The Effect of Income on Appliances in U.S. Households.* November 26, 2002.

Page 53. U.S. Department of Labor. Bureau of Labor Statistics. Consumer Expenditure Survey, 2001. *Consumer Expenditures in 2001.* April 2003.

Page 54. U.S. Department of Commerce. Economics and Statistics Administration. National Telecommunications and Information Administration. *A Nation Online: How Americans Are Expanding Their Use of the Internet.* February 2002.

Page 54. U.S. Department of Energy. Energy Information Administration. 2001 Residential Energy Consumption Survey. *The Effect of Income on Appliances in U.S. Households.* November 26, 2002.

Page 56. U.S. Department of Energy. Energy Information Administration. 2001 Residential Energy Consumption Survey. *The Effect of Income on Appliances in U.S. Households.* November 26, 2002.

Page 56. U.S. Department of Energy. Energy Information Administration. 2001 Residential Energy Consumption Survey. *The Effect of Income on Appliances in U.S. Households.* November 26, 2002.

Page 57. U.S. Department of Energy. Energy Information Administration. 2001 Residential Energy Consumption Survey. *The Effect of Income on Appliances in U.S. Households.* November 26, 2002.

Page 57. U.S. Department of Energy. Energy Information Administration. 2001 Residential Energy Consumption Survey. *The Effect of Income on Appliances in U.S. Households.* November 26, 2002.

Page 59. U.S. Department of Commerce. Economics and Statistics Administration. National Telecommunications and Information Administration. *A Nation Online: How Americans Are Expanding Their Use of the Internet.* February 2002.

Page 59. U.S. Department of Commerce. Economics and Statistics Administration. National Telecommunications and Information Administration. *A Nation Online: How Americans Are Expanding Their Use of the Internet.* February 2002.

Page 60. U.S. Department of Energy. Energy Information Administration. 2001

Residential Energy Consumption Survey. *The Effect of Income on Appliances in U.S. Households.* November 26, 2002.

Page 61. U.S. Federal Reserve Board of Governors. Federal Reserve Statistical Release. *Consumer Credit.* November 7, 2003.

Page 62. National Automobile Dealers Association (NADA). *2003 NADA Data.*

Page 63. U.S. Federal Reserve Board of Governors. Federal Reserve Statistical Release. *Consumer Credit.* November 7, 2003.

Page 65. U.S. Federal Reserve Board of Governors. Federal Reserve Statistical Release. *Consumer Credit.* November 7, 2003.

Page 67. U.S. Department of Transportation. Federal Highway Administration. *Highway Statistics 2001.* October 2002.

Page 69. U.S. Department of Transportation. Federal Highway Administration. *Highway Statistics 2001.* October 2002.

Page 69. U.S. Department of Transportation. Federal Highway Administration. *Highway Statistics 2001.* October 2002.

Page 71. U.S. Department of Commerce. U.S. Census Bureau. Census 2000. *American FactFinder.*

Page 72. U.S. Department of Commerce. U.S. Census Bureau. Census 2000. *American FactFinder.*

Page 72. U.S. Department of Transportation. Federal Highway Administration. *Highway Statistics 2001.* October 2002.

Page 73. U.S. Department of Commerce. U.S. Census Bureau. Census 2000. *American FactFinder.*

Page 76. U.S. Department of Commerce. U.S. Census Bureau. Census 2000. *American FactFinder.*

Page 77. Dr. Ing. h.c. F. Porsche AG. Official Company Website *www.porsche. com.* December 2003.

Page 78. National Automobile Dealers Association (NADA). *2003 NADA Data.*

Page 80. National Automobile Dealers Association (NADA). *2003 NADA Data.*

Page 80. U.S. Department of Transportation. Federal Highway Administration. *Highway Statistics 2001.* October 2002.

Page 82. U.S. Department of Transportation. Federal Highway Administration. *Highway Statistics 2001.* October 2002.

Page 82. National Automobile Dealers Association (NADA). *2003 NADA Data.*

Page 84. National Automobile Dealers Association (NADA). *2003 NADA Data.*

Page 85. Association of Consumer Vehicle Lessors. "Lease Volume Down

Another 7% in 2002." August 26, 2003.

Page 87. Association of Consumer Vehicle Lessors. "Lease Volume Down Another 7% in 2002." August 26, 2003.

Page 87. Association of Consumer Vehicle Lessors. "Lease Volume Down Another 7% in 2002." August 26, 2003.

Page 89. Association of Consumer Vehicle Lessors. "Lease Volume Down Another 7% in 2002." August 26, 2003.

Page 90. U.S. Department of Commerce. U.S. Census Bureau. Census 2000. *American FactFinder.*

Page 91. U.S. Department of Commerce. U.S. Census Bureau. Census 2000. *American FactFinder.*

Page 92. U.S. Department of Commerce. U.S. Census Bureau. Census 2000. *American FactFinder.*

Page 93. U.S. Department of Transportation. National Highway Traffic Safety Administration. National Center for Statistics and Analysis. *Traffic Safety Facts 2002.*

Page 95. U.S. Department of Transportation. Federal Highway Administration. *Highway Statistics 2001.* October 2002.

Page 95. U.S. Department of Transportation. Federal Highway Administration. *Highway Statistics 2001.* October 2002.

Page 96. U.S. Department of Transportation. National Highway Traffic Safety Administration. National Center for Statistics and Analysis. *Traffic Safety Facts 2002.*

Page 97. U.S. Department of Transportation. Federal Highway Administration. *Highway Statistics 2001.* October 2002.

Page 99. U.S. Department of Transportation. Federal Highway Administration. *Highway Statistics 2001.* October 2002.

Page 100. National Automobile Dealers Association (NADA). *2003 NADA Data.*

Page 100. National Automobile Dealers Association (NADA). *2003 NADA Data.*

Page 103. U.S. Department of Health and Human Services. Centers for Disease Control and Prevention. National Center for Health Statistics. *Health, United States, 2003.* September 2003.

Page 104. U.S. Department of Health and Human Services. Centers for Disease Control and Prevention. National Center for Health Statistics. *Health, United States, 2003.* September 2003.

Page 106. U.S. Department of Health and Human Services. Centers for Disease Control and Prevention. National Center for Health Statistics. *Health, United States, 2003.* September 2003.

Page 106. U.S. Department of Health and Human Services. Centers for Disease Control and Prevention. National Center for Health Statistics. *Health, United States, 2003.* September 2003.

Page 107. U.S. Department of Health and Human Services. Centers for Disease Control and Prevention. National Center for Health Statistics. *Health, United States, 2003.* September 2003.

Page 107. U.S. Department of Health and Human Services. Centers for Disease Control and Prevention. National Center for Health Statistics. *Health, United States, 2003.* September 2003.

Page 109. U.S. Department of Health and Human Services. Centers for Disease Control and Prevention. National Center for Health Statistics. *Health, United States, 2003.* September 2003.

Page 111. U.S. Federal Reserve Board of Governors. Federal Reserve Bulletin. *The Use of Checks and Other Noncash Payment Instruments in the United States.* August 2002.

Page 112. American Bankers Association. *2003 ABA Issue Summary, ATM Fact Sheet.* January 2003.

Page 112. U.S. Federal Reserve Board of Governors. Federal Reserve Bulletin. *The Use of Checks and Other Noncash Payment Instruments in the United States.* August 2002.

Page 113. U.S. Federal Reserve Board of Governors. Federal Reserve Bulletin. *The Use of Checks and Other Noncash Payment Instruments in the United States.* August 2002.

Page 113. Federal Deposit Insurance Corporation. Division of Insurance and Research. *Twenty-Five Largest Banking Companies.* Fourth Quarter 2002.

Page 114. American Bankers Association. *2003 ABA Issue Summary, ATM Fact Sheet.* January 2003.

Page 114. American Bankers Association. *2003 ABA Issue Summary, ATM Fact Sheet.* January 2003.

Page 115. U.S. Federal Reserve Board of Governors. Federal Reserve Bulletin. *The Use of Checks and Other Noncash Payment Instruments in the United States.* August 2002.

Page 116. American Bankers Association. *2003 ABA Issue Summary, ATM Fact Sheet.* January 2003.

Page 119. U.S. Federal Reserve Board of Governors. Federal Reserve Statistical

Release. *Consumer Credit*. November 7, 2003.

Page 120. U.S. Federal Reserve Board of Governors. Federal Reserve Statistical Release. *Consumer Credit*. November 7, 2003.

Page 120. U.S. Federal Reserve Board of Governors. Federal Reserve Bulletin. *The Use of Checks and Other Noncash Payment Instruments in the United States*. August 2002.

Page 121. U.S. Federal Reserve Board of Governors. Federal Reserve Bulletin. *The Use of Checks and Other Noncash Payment Instruments in the United States*. August 2002.

Page 121. U.S. Federal Reserve Board of Governors. Federal Reserve Statistical Release. *Consumer Credit*. November 7, 2003.

Page 122. U.S. Federal Reserve Board of Governors. Federal Reserve Bulletin. *Recent Changes in U.S. Family Finances: Evidence from the 1998 and 2001 Survey of Consumer Finances*. January 2003.

Page 122. U.S. Federal Reserve Board of Governors. Federal Reserve Bulletin. *Recent Changes in U.S. Family Finances: Evidence from the 1998 and 2001 Survey of Consumer Finances*. January 2003.

Page 124. U.S. Federal Reserve Board of Governors. Federal Reserve Bank of Philadelphia. Discussion Paper. Payment Cards Center. *Credit Card Pricing Developments and Their Disclosure*. January 2003.

Page 124. U.S. Federal Reserve Board of Governors. Federal Reserve Bulletin. *Recent Changes in U.S. Family Finances: Evidence from the 1998 and 2001 Survey of Consumer Finances*. January 2003.

Page 125. U.S. Federal Reserve Board of Governors. Federal Reserve Bulletin. *The Use of Checks and Other Noncash Payment Instruments in the United States*. August 2002.

Page 125. U.S. Federal Reserve Board of Governors. Federal Reserve Bulletin. *The Use of Checks and Other Noncash Payment Instruments in the United States*. August 2002.

Page 126. U.S. Federal Reserve Board of Governors. Federal Reserve Bulletin. *The Use of Checks and Other Noncash Payment Instruments in the United States*. August 2002.

Page 126. U.S. Federal Reserve Board of Governors. Federal Reserve Bulletin. *The Use of Checks and Other Noncash Payment Instruments in the United States*. August 2002.

Page 129. U.S. Department of the Treasury. Internal Revenue Service. IRS Master File System. *IRS Data Book 2002*. May 22, 2003.

Page 130. U.S. Department of the Treasury. Internal Revenue Service. IRS

Master File System. *IRS Data Book 2002*. May 22, 2003.

Page 130. U.S. Department of the Treasury. Internal Revenue Service. IRS Master File System. *IRS Data Book 2002*. May 22, 2003.

Page 131. U.S. Department of the Treasury. Internal Revenue Service. IRS Master File System. *IRS Data Book 2002*. May 22, 2003.

Page 132. U.S. Department of the Treasury. Internal Revenue Service. IRS Master File System. *IRS Data Book 2002*. May 22, 2003.

Page 133. U.S. Department of the Treasury. Internal Revenue Service. IRS Master File System. *IRS Data Book 2002*. May 22, 2003.

Page 135. United States Postal Service. *2002 Annual Report*.

Page 137. U.S. Federal Reserve Board of Governors. Federal Reserve Bank of Philadelphia. Discussion Paper. Payment Cards Center. *Credit Card Pricing Developments and Their Disclosure*. January 2003.

Page 137. U.S. Federal Reserve Board of Governors. Federal Reserve Bulletin. *The Use of Checks and Other Noncash Payment Instruments in the United States*. August 2002.

Page 138. U.S. Federal Reserve Board of Governors. Federal Reserve Bulletin. *The Use of Checks and Other Noncash Payment Instruments in the United States*. August 2002.

Page 139. U.S. Federal Reserve Board of Governors. Federal Reserve Bank of Philadelphia. Discussion Paper. Payment Cards Center. *Credit Card Pricing Developments and Their Disclosure*. January 2003.

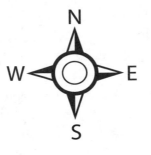

INDEX

C

REAL LIFE 101:

A GUIDE TO STUFF THAT ACTUALLY MATTERS

DEREK AVDUL
&
STEVE AVDUL

To Order Additional Copies Please Visit:

www.galtindustries.com

Or send check or money order for $15.95 plus $3.95
shipping and handling to:

Galt Industries LLC
Post Office Box 2886
Hollywood, CA 90078

For more information about the book, the authors,
or to inquire about volume discounts, please visit:

www.galtindustries.com

 GALT INDUSTRIES LLC

A MUST HAVE COMPANION!

REAL LIFE 101:
THE WORKBOOK

Create your own decision-making templates!

THE WORKBOOK provides specific worksheets tailored to every decision regarding your home, car, health, and finances including:

- Apartment Comparison Template
- Monthly Budget Calculation
- Car Leasing Versus Buying Worksheet
- Moving Checklist
- Car Payment Calculation
- Personal Finance Organizational System

This valuable tool is the only way to take the hassle out of life's everyday decisions!

To Order *Real Life 101: The Workbook* send check or money order for $6.95 plus $2.95 shipping and handling to:

Galt Industries LLC
Post Office Box 2886
Hollywood, CA 90078

or visit:
www.galtindustries.com

About The Authors

As a result of their pursuit of higher education and the demands of their chosen careers, the authors have extensive knowledge of the topics covered in this book. Collectively, they have rented over 20 separate apartments and houses in 10 cities from coast to coast. They have purchased and/or leased numerous new and used vehicles. They have been covered by health insurance from nearly a dozen different health care plans and providers. Over the years, the authors have had over 15 different bank accounts at local savings and loans, regional banks, and national financial institutions located throughout the United States. Since college, they have had literally dozens of credit cards and store charge cards from nearly every major issuer in the country.

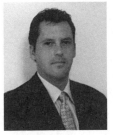

Derek Avdul has lived on his own in Oxford, OH, Hilton Head, SC, Chicago, New York, and Los Angeles. He received a Bachelor of Science in Business Administration with a concentration in marketing from Miami University (OH). Derek was also awarded a Master of Business Administration in finance from the Charles H. Kellstadt Graduate School of Business of DePaul University. Derek has worked as a market research analyst for Information Resources, Inc., a mergers and acquisitions consultant for Ernst & Young LLC, and as a director of corporate development and strategic planning for EMI Music Group. He is currently writing full time and resides in Hollywood, CA.

Steve Avdul has spent his adult life residing in Chapel Hill, NC, Philadelphia, San Francisco, Charlotte, NC, New York City, Los Angeles, and Ostersund, Sweden. Steve earned a Bachelor of Science in Business Administration from the University of North Carolina at Chapel Hill as well as a Master of Business Administration in finance from 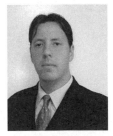 the Wharton School of the University of Pennsylvania. He has spent his entire professional career working on Wall Street in the field of private equity focusing on leveraged buyouts, most recently for Credit Suisse First Boston. Steve has traveled extensively throughout the United States and has been around the world several times visiting over 60 countries across six continents. Steve lives in New York City.